FEESST

FLEXIBLE ENDOSCOPIC EVALUATION OF SWALLOWING WITH SENSORY TESTING

Jonathan E. Aviv, MD

Thomas Murry, PhD

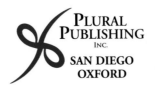

PLURAL
PUBLISHING
INC.
SAN DIEGO
OXFORD

Plural Publishing, Inc.
6256 Greenwich Drive, Suite 230
San Diego, CA 92122

London office:
49 Bath Street
Abington, Oxfordshire 0K14 1 EA
London, UK 0X14 lEA

e-mail: info@pluralpublishing.com
Web site: http://www.pluralpublishing.com

Typeset in 11/13 Palatino by So Cal Graphics
Printed in Hong Kong by Paramount Book Art, Inc.

For permission to use material from this text, contact us by
Telephone: (866) 758-7251
Fax: (888) 758-7255
www.pluralpublishing.com

Care has been taken to confirm the accuracy of the information presented in this book and to describe generally accepted practices. However, the authors, editors, and publisher are not responsible for errors or omissions or for any consequences from application of the information in this book and make no warranty, expressed or implied, with respect to the currency, completeness, or accuracy of the contents of the publication. Application of this information in a particular situation remains the professional responsibility of the practitioner.

The authors, editors, and publisher have exerted every effort to ensure that drug selection and dosage in this text are in accordance with current recommendations and practice at the time of publication. However, in view of ongoing research, changes in government regulations, and the constant flow of information on drug therapy and drug reactions, the reader is urged to check the package insert for each drug for any change in indications and dosage and for added warnings and precautions.

ISBN 1-59756-000-6
Library of Congress Control Number: 2005924391

Contents

Foreword

The patient with dysphagia presents many challenges in diagnosis and management. Traditional teaching divides this symptom into two broad components—oropharyngeal and esophageal dysphagia. The emphasis of this book is on oropharyngeal dysphagia, which often presents a greater challenge because the etiology is more often multifactorial, with abnormalities of the upper esophageal sphincter, larynx, and pharynx seen in the same patient. Structural and sensory deficits often co-exist and confound the clinician; thus, the need for a multidisciplinary approach, involving multiple specialties and diagnostic modalities. Throughout this book, the authors remind us that swallowing should be viewed as a combination of two distinct but interrelated phenomena, airway protection and bolus transport. When examining the sensory and motor aspects of swallowing, a multifaceted diagnostic approach is required combining optimal use of laryngopharyngeal sensory testing and transnasal flexible endoscopy, with a bolus challenge. When performed carefully, this comprehensive evaluation of oropharyngeal dysphagia almost always yields an accurate diagnosis, usually with a unifying single cause.

In this well-written book, Drs. Aviv and Murry provide a state-of-the-art reference source for the clinicians who are considering or already performing flexible endoscopic evaluation of swallowing with sensory testing (FEESST). All facets of the technique are carefully and clearly covered, including the evolving potential for transnasal esophagoscopy. The final chapters on coding and case studies are added highlights. For specialists involved in the evaluation and care of patients with swallowing disorders, this book offers clear, practical information on the technique and its vital role in evaluating patients with dysphagia. This "esophagologist" learned much about an area outside of my personal domain, one underap-

preciated by my specialty. I intend to have it included in our fel-
lows' curriculum. You will find it an easy but valuable read.

Philip O. Katz, MD
Professor and Chair, Division of Gastroenterology
Albert Einstein Medical Center
Philadelphia, Pennsylvania

Preface

The past 25 years have produced a tremendous growth in the field of dysphagia, or difficulty in swallowing. The old philosophy of the dysphagia workup was simply to send the patient out of the office to obtain a modified barium swallow (MBS) and then to see a speech-language pathologist (SLP) for "exercises." This philosophy of fluoroscopy first and then off to the SLP resulted in most physicians avoiding the opportunity to address a dysphagia consultation. With the advent of endoscopy for swallowing beginning in the late 1980s, laryngopharyngeal sensory testing in the early 1990s, and transnasal esophagoscopy in the late 1990s, physician interest in swallowing disorders has accelerated dramatically. Along with this growing physician interest in dysphagia diagnosis and treatment has come a concomitant appreciation of the importance of physicians working together with SLPs to comprehensively care for the patient with dysphagia. SLPs continue to remain largely responsible for the rehabilitation of swallowing disorders.

Indeed, what has happened is that, through research and clinical care, clinicians from many disciplines have identified a broad range of individuals with an extensive array of swallowing disorders. These disorders are seen in patients after a stroke, those with chronic neurodegenerative disease, and individuals after head and neck cancer surgery, cardiac surgery, and other surgeries during which the aerodigestive tract has been manipulated. In addition, clinicians have seen an increase in the number of relatively healthy patients who are searching for the reason that they feel a continuous lump in their throat that interferes with swallowing.

As an otolaryngologist–head and neck surgeon and as a speech-language pathologist, we have been combining our experiences and areas of expertise in sensory testing, fiberoptic endoscopic evaluation of swallowing (FEES), and flexible endoscopic evaluation of swallowing with sensory testing (FEESST), both separately and together, over the past decade. Due to the nature of our practices, we began to see a broad range of patients with swallowing complaints. Many of them were referred from colleagues who felt more specific tests and different treatments were needed to improve the problems that remained after first-line treatment. Together, we developed a unique clinical approach using specific case history forms, patient examination techniques, and diagnostic tests to reach a diagnosis and offer a plan of treatment.

This text brings together in one volume a relatively new series of tests—sensory testing, FEES, and FEESST. It is the first text that provides the history of sensory testing, the rationale for sensory testing, and the role of sensory testing in patients with a broad range of voice and swallowing complaints. Central to the diagnosis and management of swallowing is a thorough knowledge of the anatomy, physiology, and neurophysiology of normal swallowing. Therefore, we present a detailed understanding of swallowing in Chapter I. Emphasis is on the normal anatomy of the head and neck as it relates to swallowing.

The following two chapters present the FEESST technique itself and how it applies to specific populations such as the elderly and those who have had a stroke. Chapter IV describes sensory testing as a stand-alone test without a complete assessment of swallowing to permit the type of evaluation necessary to fully evaluate laryngopharyngeal acid reflux disease as well as laryngopharyngeal sensory function. The importance of asymmetric and symmetric sensory thresholds and their implications for diagnosis are discussed.

In Chapter V, we present an extension of normal swallow assessment, transnasal esophagoscopy (TNE). This area of testing is becoming increasingly more important because of the astonishing rise of esophageal cancer. Because of its use as an office-based examination, this technique, and its implications, are relevant not only to otolaryngologists, but also to all clinicians involved in the care of esophageal disease.

Chapter VI delves into the details of how safe FEESST is to perform. In Chapter VII, we turn to the practical aspect of sensory testing and swallowing evaluations, that is, diagnostic and procedure coding. We have been integrally involved with the development of coding for each of the examinations described in this book and share that experience as it will likely serve as a blueprint for how to handle the inevitable changes that will take place in the coding system.

The book concludes with the presentation of several representative cases from our clinical experience with sensory testing and FEESST. Although this group of cases is not exhaustive, the reader will obtain a broad-based understanding of the rationale leading to specific tests and treatment planning.

The diagnosis and treatment of swallowing disorders has been established as an interdisciplinary task in previous texts. Specialists whose research and clinical practice concentrate on diseases of the head and neck, gastrointestinal tract, lungs, heart, brain, and nervous system will find the application of sensory testing along with the functional assessment of swallowing disorders to be an essential step in the overall rehabilitation of patients. With this book, we offer a practical, yet specialized, approach to the management of laryngopharyngeal sensory disorders and dysphagia.

Jonathan E. Aviv, MD
Thomas Murry, PhD

List of Commonly Appearing Abbreviations

ALS—amyotrophic lateral sclerosis (Lou Gherig's disease)

CMS—Center for Medicaid and Medicare Services

CN—cranial nerve

CPT—current procedural terminology

CP—cricopharyngeus

CT—computerized tomography

CVA—cerebrovascular accident

EG—esophagogastric

EGD—esophagogastroduodenoscopy

EMG—electromyography

FEES—fiberoptic endoscopic evaluation of swallowing

FEESST—flexible endoscopic evaluation of swallowing with sensory testing

GE—gastroesophageal

GERD—gastroesophageal reflux disease

GI—gastrointestinal

H2—histamine two

ICU—intensive care unit

LAR—laryngeal adductor reflex

LES—lower esophageal sphincter

LPR—laryngopharyngeal reflux

MBS—modified barium swallow

MRI—magnetic resonance imaging

PEG—percutaneous endoscopic gastrostomy

PPI—proton pump inhibitor

RFS—reflux finding score

RLN—recurrent laryngeal nerve

RSI—reflux symptom index

RVU—relative value unit

SLN—superior laryngeal nerve

SLP—speech-language pathologist

TE—transesophageal echocardiography

TFL—transnasal flexible laryngoscopy

TIA—transient ischemic attack

TNE—transnasal esophagoscopy

UES—upper esophageal sphincter

URI—upper respiratory infection

VHI 10—Voice Handicap Index (10 Questions)

Dedication

To the inspiration of Caleigh, Nikki, and Blake.

To Marie-Pierre and Nicholas for their support and trust.

I

Introduction to Swallowing

1. Why FEESST?
2. Structure of the Voice and Swallowing Center
3. Importance of dysphagia
4. Endoscopic anatomy
5. Swallowing physiology
6. Summary

1. WHY FEESST?

Swallowing is a complex process that involves an interplay between two distinct but related phenomena, airway protection and bolus transport.[1] Almost all tests of swallowing—videofluoroscopy or modified barium swallow (MBS), barium swallow or esophagram, fiberoptic endoscopic examination of swallowing (FEES)— look specifically at bolus transport and ignore or infer airway protective capacity. Early research on transnasal flexible endoscopy for swallowing suggested the importance of sensitivity testing of the larynx during an endoscopic swallowing evaluation. What these early works described was touching or tapping the laryngopharyngeal tissues with the tip of the endoscope and assessing the patient's reaction to such stimulation.[2,3] Touching or tapping tissues with an endoscope tip is an extremely subjective way to assess sensory capacity. Questions arise such as: How much tapping is necessary? How forceful should the tap be? What part of the laryngopharynx should be tapped? What reaction is the clinician looking for? Will clinicians tap the same way, in the same location, from one time to the next? Moreover, movement of the endoscope itself may cause a reaction prior to tapping the tissues. Furthermore, it is difficult to translate the reaction to a tissue tap from one patient to another and from the same patient one day to the same patient 3 months from now.

Flexible endoscopic evaluation of swallowing with sensory testing (FEESST) is the only test of a swallow that examines both airway protection and bolus transport. Airway protection is determined by administering a calibrated pressure and duration-controlled pulse of air to the hypopharyngeal tissues innervated by the internal branch of the superior laryngeal nerve (SLN) in order to elicit the laryngeal adductor reflex (LAR), a fundamental, brainstem-mediated airway protective reflex.[4] It has been shown that the afferent signal arising from the internal branch of the SLN is necessary for normal deglutition, especially for providing feedback to central neural circuits that facilitate laryngeal adduction during swallowing.[5]

The following clinical scenario brings into immediate focus the importance of sensory testing in directing the management of patients with dysphagia:

A physician is called to see a 68-year-old man in the intensive care unit, who is complaining of dysphagia 3 days after his open heart surgery and is currently not taking food by mouth. An MBS and a FEES examination are performed the same day, and each test demonstrates minor laryngeal penetration and slight aspiration.

With this information, the clinician must now decide how to manage this patient. Does the clinician recommend that the patient be given food by mouth or that the patient be kept on non-oral alimentation? What would you do?

The fact is, with the information given so far, it is virtually impossible to know whether or not to feed the patient. Usually, the clinician will use other information, such as general health of the patient, discharge planning, and so forth, to make the decision. In essence, the results of the instrumental tests are not involved in the decision-making process.

However, if the same patient, with the same swallowing test result, had a laryngeal sensory test prior to the administration of food with the flexible endoscope in situ (a FEESST examination), and the test showed that the patient was able to protect his airway (ie, he had an intact LAR or normal laryngopharyngeal sensory thresholds), then one would—with great confidence—feed the patient despite the slight aspiration. On the other hand, if the laryngeal sensory test on this patient showed an absent LAR bilaterally (indicating a bilateral, severe sensory deficit), the patient would not be given food by mouth, because the patient has significant impairment of his airway protective reflexes. Using this information, the clinician would feel confident in reporting that this patient is at high risk for aspiration. With information obtained from the FEESST regarding both the patient's sensory and motor functions, the patient with aspiration is managed quite differently depending on what his sensory test results show. The sensory test, along with the food administration portion of the FEESST, provides comprehensive information regarding both sensory and motor functions of the swallowing mechanism. Neither FEES nor MBS alone allows the clinician to safely make a decision to feed the patient.

In the following sections of this chapter, we describe how we have set up our voice and swallowing center, and explain why dysphagia is important to study and treat. The remainder of the chapter consists of a detailed description of the endoscopic anatomy of the head and neck and its application to understanding swallowing physiology.

2. STRUCTURE OF THE VOICE AND SWALLOWING CENTER

Philosophy and Personnel

There are many ways to set up a voice and swallowing center. We believe that the essential components can be broadly divided into personnel and equipment categories. Our philosophical preference is to develop a center where communication between clinicians and patient is ongoing and direct. Thus, using this model, the key members are in close proximity and interact in the testing and treatment phases of patient care.

Personnel requirements start with an otolaryngologist–head and neck surgeon and a speech-language pathologist. At the Voice and Swallowing Center at Columbia University College of Physicians & Surgeons at New York-Presbyterian Hospital, all patients are seen simultaneously by an otolaryngologist and a speech-language pathologist. The rationale for having two "swallowologists" with different professional backgrounds concomitantly seeing the same patient and the same test is that this combination of the medical diagnostic aspect and nonsurgical therapeutic aspect of swallowing disorders provides unparalleled continuity of care for the patient. Although the digital or analog media of a particular swallowing examination can serve the purpose of the therapeutic team seeing the "same things," nothing is as complete and efficient as the shared real-time experience of the physical examination.

Physicians and other health care professionals with specific areas of expertise are integral for the comprehensive care of patients at our center. In particular, the following physician specialties are necessary: gastroenterology, pulmonology, neurology, physiatry, and radiology. Nonphysician health care professionals are also vitally important to completely care for our patients; they include nurses, registered dieticians, and social workers. How these different areas of expertise are woven together to care for our patients is illustrated with the following example:

> A 49-year-old practicing accountant who is otherwise healthy and is on no prescription medications is seen in the Voice and Swallowing Center. He was referred by his internist for an assessment of swallowing-related complaints. The patient reports a 6-month history of waxing and wan-

ing right-sided searing throat pain, frequent throat clearing, a lumplike sensation in his throat, intermittent cough not related to eating, occasional shortness of breath, and a 10 lb weight loss. The patient also notes periodic nausea when eating a "spicy" meal, although he denies heartburn ("I never get heartburn, by the way, what is heartburn?"). The patient is unsure if he had an upper respiratory infection prior to symptom onset.

On physical examination, tongue fasciculations are noted. The laryngeal structures are visualized with a transnasal flexible laryngoscope, and normal vocal fold mobility is observed with no vocal fold lesions. There is evidence of pseudosulcus vocalis, partial ventricle obliteration, and arytenoid and interarytenoid edema. No pooling of secretions in piriform sinuses is noted at the onset of the examination.

Laryngopharyngeal sensory testing reveals a severe right-sided laryngeal sensory deficit and normal laryngeal sensory thresholds on the left. Following sensory testing, the vocal folds are seen to be adducting to more than 50% of the glottic airway during quiet respiration. Moreover, after a swallow, the vocal folds remain completely adducted for 1 to 2 seconds. The adductory motion of the vocal folds suggests paradoxic vocal fold motion along with a unilateral sensory deficit.

The patient's diagnoses thus far are laryngopharyngeal reflux (LPR) (frequent throat clearing, globus sensation, signs of LPR on the flexible laryngoscopy part of sensory testing); right SLN pathology (searing right-sided throat pain, asymmetric sensory testing results—maybe neuropathy, maybe neuralgia); and paradoxic vocal fold motion disorder (cough, vocal folds closing when they should be opening).

This examination poses several interesting questions. How do the tongue fasciculations play a role here? How does this information get sorted out in preparation for a treatment plan? Are the otolaryngologist and the speech-language pathologist the only health care professionals this patient needs to solve his problems?

Step by step, the outcome of this examination results in the comprehensive management by several individuals, each with a specific role. We suggest a management plan by the following individuals:

Gastroenterology: An upper GI endoscopy is necessary to rule out gastric pathology (nausea complaint) and Barrett esophagus (LPR diagnosis). Esophageal manometry and motility testing would be helpful as well.

Pulmonology: Spirometry with analysis of flow volume loops is necessary to determine the contribution of pulmonary dysfunction to the shortness of breath complaint.

Neurology: Rule out subtle, early chronic neurodegenerative disease (tongue fasciculations).

Physiatry: Pain management may be necessary if this turns out to be a neuralgia of some sort.

Radiology: Imaging of the brain, neck, and upper mediastinum is necessary to rule out central or peripheral pathology along the course of the right vagus nerve and right SLN.

Dietitian: A calorie count is needed to determine what the patient's caloric requirements are and what he needs to sustain himself with oral intake alone.

With information provided by each of these specialists, a goal-directed management program can be initiated. The swallowing center personnel will maintain complete records of each test and coordinate the patient's ongoing treatment and follow-up sensory testing and swallowing evaluations.

Equipment in the Voice and Swallowing Center

What equipment is essential for a voice and swallowing center? The basic instrumentation for a general otolaryngology office includes headlights, nasal speculae, tongue depressors, and topical anesthetics and decongestants. Digital or analog recording capability is also required. Video hardware and software with adequate archiving capability are also necessary in an active swallowing center so that access to past examinations is rapid. Flexible and rigid endoscopes for access to the laryngopharynx and esophagus are vital as well and are detailed in chapter II. In addition, a stroboscope is essential. The radiology equipment is not critical to have on site, but is helpful. Once the center's personnel and equipment are set, the patient with dysphagia can be assessed and treated in a systematic fashion.

3. IMPORTANCE OF DYSPHAGIA

Dysphagia, the inability to swallow normally and its sequelae, is an extremely common clinical condition that affects millions of people annually in all age groups. By examining incidence of dysphagia following a stroke, one can begin to grasp the enormity of the dysphagia problem. Approximately 500,000 people per year in the United States have a stroke with up to 65% of these patients experiencing some type of swallowing difficulty.[6,7] It is not the acute neurologic injury after stroke that usually causes patient demise; rather, the pulmonary complications after stroke, in particular aspiration pneumonia, are deadly. There are many reasons poststroke patients develop aspiration pneumonia; however, dysphagia and its consequences are a primary source of the additional morbidity and possibly mortality after a stroke.[7] Difficulty in swallowing results in the inability to handle safely what one eats and drinks. As a result, some of what one eats or secretes may enter the lungs, which in turn precipitates severe pulmonary infections.

The real problem with aspiration pneumonia after stroke is not that an isolated pneumonia takes place. The wrenching fact is that aspiration pneumonia is an annuity of progressive debilitation for the patient, placing the patient in a spiraling decrease of general health. Recurrent aspiration pneumonia, in some cases rapidly and in other cases slowly over a several year period, leads to an overall reduction in quality of life and decreased health status until the patient finally succumbs.[8] The recurrent episodes of aspiration pneumonia are what the dysphagia diagnostic testing team must be aware of and alert to when treating stroke patients.

An examination of what has been happening to the chronic care population capsulizes the "circling of the drain" that takes place as a result of aspiration pneumonia. Pneumonia as a result of recurrent aspiration of food and secretions is the most likely reason for residents of chronic care facilities to be discharged from their facility and sent to a hospital.[9,10] Furthermore, the attack rate for pneumonia is highest among those in nursing homes.[11] Thirty-three of every 1,000 nursing home residents per year required hospitalization for treatment of pneumonia, as compared with 1.14 of 1000 elderly adults living in an open community.[10]

Once the nursing home patient enters or re-enters the hospital for treatment of pneumonia, costs escalate dramatically. The annual health care cost in the United States for treating aspiration pneumonia in the nursing home population alone is estimated to be $4.4 billion.[12-14] As the population ages, aspiration pneumonia will have an even greater impact on health care costs.[15]

To make a dent in the numbers of patients suffering from aspiration pneumonia, the clinician must be able to make an accurate diagnosis of the patient with dysphagia so that a tailored therapy can be administered. The diagnostic focus should be on determining if the patient can maintain adequate caloric oral intake of food and liquid, not on whether or not a droplet of barium or applesauce has traversed the vocal folds. The overriding reason for examining patients with swallowing difficulties is to determine if it is safe for them to swallow. Only after that should management strategies be considered.

4. ENDOSCOPIC ANATOMY

A thorough familiarity with the endoscopic anatomy of the nasal cavity, nasopharynx, oropharynx, and hypopharynx is essential to the successful performance and interpretation of a FEESST. All of the endoscopic images of the hypopharynx in this book will have the same orientation with the base of tongue and anterior portion of the larynx located along the inferior aspect of the image and the esophageal inlet and posterior portion of the larynx oriented along the superior aspect of the image (Fig 1–1).

Nasal Anatomy

Three structures in the nose have to be examined to ensure safe, unobstructed passage of the flexible endoscope from the nose into the oropharynx: the nasal septum, inferior turbinate, and middle turbinate (Fig 1–2). Certain variations in normal anatomy may make transnasal passage of the endoscope difficult. Nasal septal deviations are a very common cause of unilateral nasal obstruction (Fig 1–3). Generally, if one side of the nose has a very deviated septum, the other side will be more patent and allow for unobstructed scope passage. Another septal variation that is relatively common and can be confusing to the endoscopist is a nasal septal perforation (Fig 1–4). Care must be taken not to inadvertently traverse the opening in the perforated septum, because such a maneuver likely will make it difficult to readily advance the endoscope, as well as possibly cause nasal septal trauma resulting in epistaxis, or nosebleed. Another common pathological condition of the nasal cavity is nasal polyps, which can cause significant nasal obstruction (Fig 1–5). Despite these variations in normal endoscopic anatomy, it is

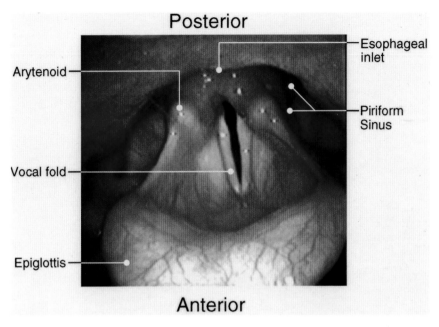

FIGURE 1-1. Endoscopic appearance of the hypopharynx in a healthy patient. The cartilaginous facets of the paired arytenoid cartilages are readily visualized.

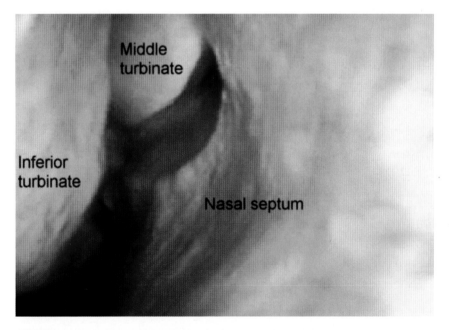

FIGURE 1-2. Endoscopic appearance of right nasal cavity. The right middle turbinate effectively lies between the nasal septum on one side and the right inferior turbinate on the other side.

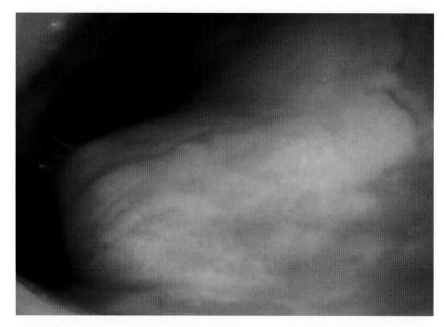

FIGURE 1–3. Right nasal septal deviation. There is a large nasal septal spur jutting into the right nasal cavity as part of a deviated nasal septum to the right.

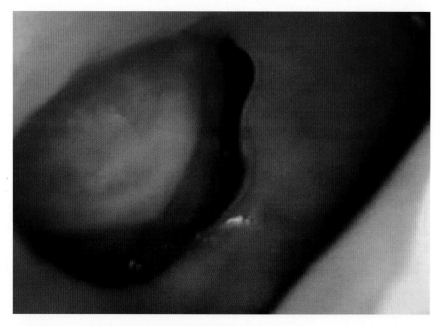

FIGURE 1–4. Nasal septal perforation. This is an endoscopic view of the left nasal cavity. The right inferior turbinate is visualized through a rather large hole in the nasal septum. Normally, one would not be able to see any right nasal cavity structures when endoscopically examining the left side of the nose.

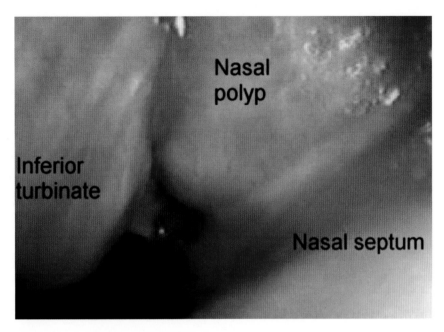

FIGURE 1–5. Right nasal polyp. Endoscopic view within the right nasal cavity. The right nasal polyp is a fleshy mass squeezed between the right inferior turbinate and the nasal septum.

well established that FEESST is extremely safe. (Swallowing safety will be discussed in Chapter VI.)

Nasopharynx, Oropharynx, and Hypopharynx

The key structure to pay attention to in the nasopharynx is the taurus tubaris which is the anatomic landmark representing the eustachian tube opening into the nasopharynx (Fig 1–6). After the scope is passed through the nasopharynx, the base of the tongue, valeculla, and supraglottic structures are encountered. In patients with a dysphagia complaint, a detailed endoscopic inspection of the tongue base and valeculla should take place as base of tongue tumors can be detected during this portion of a transnasal flexible laryngoscopy (TFL).

Subsequent to inspection of the tongue base, inspection of the larynx should take place. Attention should be focused on the presence or absence of laryngeal masses. In addition, symmetry of the vocal folds and arytenoids should be observed. The interarytenoid tissue and the posterior commissure should be noted for presence

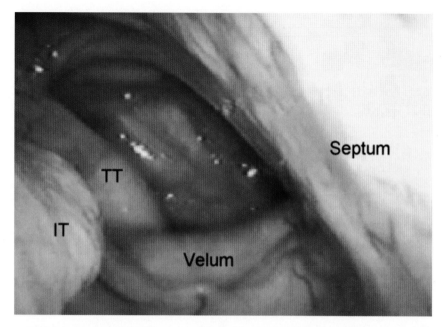

FIGURE 1–6. Taurus tubaris. Endoscopic view within the right nasal cavity. The taurus tubaris (*TT*) is located in the nasopharynx just posterior to the edge of the velum, or soft palate. Note the right inferior turbinate (*IT*).

of edema. The presence of vocal fold immobility should be noted as well. The reason a visual assessment of laryngeal motion should take place in a patient with a dysphagia complaint is that impaired vocal fold mobility, especially in abduction, could herald a vagal mass or a neoplasm in the skull base, neck, or mediastinum. In addition to assessment of vocal fold mobility, a detailed assessment of vocal fold anatomy should take place. In particular, the presence of signs of acid reflux disease should be documented. The acid reflux signs to pay particular attention to are the presence of pseudosulcus vocalis, ventricle obliteration, arytenoid and interarytenoid edema, and posterior commissure hypertrophy (Fig 1–7). As will be discussed in Chapter IV, sensory testing can quantify the degree of posterior laryngeal swelling that results from chronic acid reflux injury to the arytenoid and interarytenoid regions.

Once the larynx is visualized, the piriform sinuses should be identified. These paired cone-shaped structures lying on either side of the endolarynx serve as the gateway to the esophageal inlet of the postcricoid region (see Fig 1–1). Especially, it should be noted whether or not excess fluids or saliva are seen in these areas.

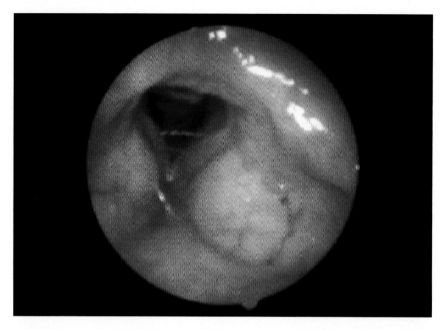

FIGURE 1-7. The endoscopic stigmata of laryngopharyngeal reflux. This patient had absolutely no complaints of heartburn or regurgitation, but rather was complaining of hoarseness, cough, throat clearing, and increased phlegm. Note the pseudosulcus vocalis, which is subglottic edema, seen better under the left true vocal fold. Also seen is ventricle obliteration—the space between the true and false vocal fold that should be 1 to 2 mm, but is obliterated in this image. In addition, there is arytenoid and interarytenoid edema as well as thick endolaryngeal mucus. Note the bridges of thick mucus sitting across the vocal folds.

5. SWALLOWING PHYSIOLOGY

The anatomic structures of the oral cavity, nasopharynx, oropharynx, and hypopharynx work to produce a normal swallow as a result of the sensory, motor, and temporal integration of the anatomy just reviewed. But what is happening physiologically?

A normal and safe transport of food or liquid from the lips to the stomach requires the combined activity of the sensory and motor components of the swallowing organs. This sensory-motor integration traditionally has been separated into four phases: (1) oral preparatory phase, (2) oral phase, (3) pharyngeal phase, and (4) esophageal phase.[16] Others have chosen to consider swallowing in three phases, oral, pharyngeal, and esophageal, with the oral phase having two distinct divisions, the oral preparatory and the oral transport phases.[17] The oral phase of swallowing is under voluntary control, whereas the pharyngeal and esophageal phases represent a complex set of neuromuscular controls. Although it is convenient to describe involuntary swallowing according to three or four phases, it should be remembered that these phases are not isolated stages but rather are interactive.

Oral Phase

The oral phase of swallowing consists of preparing the bolus for transport and then transporting it from the oral cavity to the oropharynx. In the first part of the oral phase, sometimes called the oral preparatory phase, food or liquid enters the oral cavity. Lip closure occurs to contain the bolus, and the tongue and mandible are activated to move the bolus to the teeth for mastication. Mastication involves normal motion of the tongue, mandible, and teeth combined with saliva to aid in the preparation of the bolus for the next phase.[18] During feeding and mastication, the anterior two-thirds of the tongue is critical for bolus formation and movement. In addition, at the same time, the velum, elevated by the tensor and levator palatini muscles and the palatopharyngeus muscles provide a seal to the nasopharynx to prevent food or liquids from entering the nasal cavity. While this phase of swallowing continues, respiration is generally ongoing. Thus, it is possible that small bits of food or liquids may escape the oral cavity into the oropharynx, esophagus, or trachea causing an individual to cough or choke while masticating. The final act of the oral preparatory phase is a series of movements of the tongue and mandible to locate the bolus on the tongue in anticipation of the bolus transport phase.

Once the bolus has completed the preparatory phase in the oral cavity, it is ready for transport. The velum is elevated, as described above, and the tongue depresses posteriorly. The anterior and middle thirds of the tongue elevate with pressure against the hard palate moving the bolus to the oropharynx. Kahrilas et al described centripetal and centrifugal motions of the posterior tongue to propel the bolus in the posterior direction.[19] The oral transit phase, which is highly dependent on the posterior one-third of the tongue, channels the bolus to the faucial arches. If done in proper temporal sequence, the bolus is now ready for the pharyngeal phase of swallowing.

Oral Phase Innervation

Normal tongue musculature is essential in the oral phase of swallowing. Aviv summarized the contributions of the extrinsic and intrinsic tongue muscles active during swallowing.[20] The extrinsic muscles consist of the genioglossus, hyoglossus, styloglossus, and palatopharyngeus. Their insertions are either to the hyoid bone (hyoglossus) or interlacing into other extrinsic or intrinsic tongue muscles at various locations in the tongue. For swallowing, the extrinsic muscles serve primarily to position the tongue according to the action required, either anterior/posterior or upward/downward.

Intrinsic tongue musculature produces changes in the shape of the tongue during mastication and transport. The longitudinal, vertical, and transverse tongue muscles have no bony attachments. Their insertions are to each other and to the extrinsic muscles of the tongue.

Both the sensory and motor systems of the tongue contribute to the normal oral phase of swallowing. The primary afferent control of the tongue as well as the lips and mandible is via cranial nerve (CN) V. Efferent control of the tongue is via CN XII, whereas CN VII controls efferent activity of the lips, and CNs V, VII, and X control the motor activity of the mandible.

CN V contains both sensory and motor fibers. The sensory fibers in the mandibular division send impulses from the anterior two-thirds of the tongue, cheek, and floor of the mouth primarily to the nuclei in the upper midbrain.[21] Fibers from the primary sensory nuclei terminate in the ventral posterior medial nucleus of the thalamus. Efferent stimulation of the tongue is via CN XII. This nerve serves the longitudinal (superior and inferior) transverse and vertical intrinsic muscles of the tongue as well as the extrinsic muscles, namely the hyoglossus and genioglossus muscles.

During the oral phase of swallowing, there is continuous interaction of the tongue and mandible. While the intrinsic and extrinsic muscles activate the tongue, the orbicularis oris, buccinator, and, primarily, the lateral pterygoid muscles are responsible for controlling the motion of the lips, cheek, and mandible.[22] Remarkably, all of the afferent and efferent interactions of the oral phase of swallowing generally take about 1 second to complete. However, duration of the oral phase of swallowing varies not only with age, but also with sensory awareness, type of bolus, and health of the individual.[23]

Pharyngeal Phase

Once the bolus is masticated, reformed into a semisolid consistency in the case of food, and then positioned on the tongue, it is ready to be merged into the pharyngeal phase of swallowing. The actions during the pharyngeal phase are under involuntary neuromuscular control. The mouth is usually closed to allow pressure to build up to pump the bolus posteriorly and inferiorly into the oropharynx. At the same time, the velum makes contact with the posterior pharyngeal wall to seal off the nasal cavity. When a patient reports nasal regurgitation, the velum should be observed during the strong production of /k,k,k/ to assess velar movement. Velar elevation is accomplished by contraction of the palatopharyngeus sphincter (levator veli palatini muscles) and, to some extent, part of the superior constrictor muscle.[24] Although the uvula may vary in size, there has been no evidence to show that size alone has any effect on its ability to achieve closure of the nasal cavity during deglutition.

The pharyngeal phase is thought to begin when the bolus passes the anterior faucial arches. At the same time, there is posterior movement of the tongue carrying the bolus toward the oropharynx. This is accompanied by sensory stimulation to the pharynx, which is thought to contribute to the movement of the bolus.[25] Pharyngeal sensation has been shown to play a key role during this portion of the pharyngeal phase of swallowing. Ludlow et al demonstrated effective action of the swallow reflex with direct stimulation to the internal branch of the SLN.[26] As mentioned earlier, it has been shown that a 50-millisecond (ms) air pulse to the mucosa innervated by the SLN results in a laryngeal adductor response in normal individuals.[4]

The events that follow or coincide with velopharyngeal closure occur in rapid succession. The vocal folds adduct, the hyoid bone elevates, and a "pumplike" motion of the oral structures occurs. This is coupled with the opening of the upper esophageal sphincter, which creates a pressure differential across the hypopharynx with the higher pressure from the oral cavity pushing the bolus into an opening of lower air pressure in the esophagus. The superior pharyngeal constrictor has also been shown to have a reflexive function that contributes to laryngeal elevation and hyoid advancement. The pressure pump results from closure of the lips and velopharynx coupled with the action of the buccal muscles and elevation of the tongue to the hard palate. McConnel et al studied the motion of the food bolus during the onset of the pharyngeal phase using pharyngeal pressure sensors and videoflouroscopy.[27] He described two pumps, the oropharyngeal propulsion pump and the hypopharyngeal suction pump. The oropharyngeal propulsion pump is created by the lips, cheeks, and tongue and serves as the driving pressure for the food bolus. The hypopharyngeal suction pump is created by the negative pressure that results when the cricopharyngeus muscle (CP) snaps open and laryngeal elevation occurs, which then serves as a clearing force for the bolus. McConnel's results are further evidence that there is complementary action between the oral and the pharyngeal phases of swallowing.

Propulsion of the bolus leads to vocal fold adduction and elevation of the hyoid and larynx.[28,29] The elevation action of the hyoid and larynx, along with closure of the vocal folds, creates the primary protection from aspiration. The epiglottis, although not the primary source of airway protection, can be thought of as a weathervane of sensory protection because the greatest concentration of sensory nerve fibers occurs at the tip of the epiglottis.[30] Additional protection is offered by the adduction of the false vocal folds. The retroflexive motion of the epiglottis, although not the primary source of airway protection, serves partially as a funnel to direct the bolus posteriorly and laterally toward the piriform sinuses.

Vocal fold closure during each swallow necessarily implies a period of apnea. This means that the individual is not breathing during each swallow for a specific time period usually ranging between 0.3 to 2.5 seconds. For patients with neuromuscular disorders or those with compromised pulmonary capacity, these repeated instances of "forced apnea" during every swallow result in an insidious fatigue of the airway's protective capacity. As a result, during the progression of a meal, patients are at higher and higher risk for aspiration.[31]

What makes this situation so dangerous is that, at the beginning of a meal or the beginning of a modified barium swallow, these patients do not show aspiration; and the clinician is given a false-negative study, which can be life-threatening. One of the key features of FEESST is that, because X-rays are not involved, the clinician has the time to see fatigue during a meal and then make the appropriate safety recommendations. Once the bolus is in motion by the oropharyngeal and hypopharyngeal pump actions, it is moved farther along by contraction of the middle and inferior pharyngeal constrictors, leading to the esophageal phase.

Pharyngeal Phase Innervation

Both sensory and motor controls are active in the pharyngeal phase of swallowing, as they are in the oral phase. The sensory control of the pharyngeal phase is governed in large part by the SLN. As early as 1953, Ogura and Lam demonstrated laryngeal closure and swallowing movements using electrical stimulation of the SLN in animals and humans.[32] Later, Aviv et al demonstrated SLN reflexive activity by using an air pressure stimulus to the aryepiglottic folds that resulted in adductory motion of the arytenoids.[33]

A recent study of the SLN by Jafari et al suggested that damage to the SLN alone, without additional airway or brain lesions, can result in dysphagia and aspiration.[5] Moreover, based on their research, they suggested that SLN damage is a major factor for dysphagia and aspiration following conservative laryngeal surgery.

In the pharyngeal phase of swallowing, afferent control of the tongue base, the lingual surface of the epiglottis, and the oro- and nasopharynx is by CN IX, the glossopharyngeal nerve. This nerve sends touch, pain, and thermal stimulation from the posterior third of the tongue and from the mucous membranes of the oropharynx and faucial pillars. Efferent action of CN IX results in contraction of the stylopharyngeus muscle to elevate the pharynx.

CN X, the vagus nerve, may be considered the primary motor and sensory control system for normal and safe swallowing. The internal branch of the SLN is responsible for sensation from the laryngeal surface of the epiglottis and laryngopharynx to the level of the vocal folds. The recurrent laryngeal nerve (RLN) contributes sensory information below the vocal folds and the esophagus. The pharyngeal branch of the vagus nerve contributes sensory information from the levator palatini and superior and middle constrictors.[34] Finally, the esophageal branch of CN X conveys sensory information from the mucosa and striated muscles of the esophagus. Together, these afferent systems of the CN X provide awareness of sensation and taste.

The recurrent laryngeal branch of the CN X controls laryngeal closure through all of the intrinsic muscles of the larynx except the posterior cricoarytenoid. The recurrent branch activates the thyroarytenoid, thyroepiglottic, lateral cricoarytenoids, transverse arytenoids, and oblique arytenoids. The posterior cricoarytenoid muscle, also controlled by CN X, is the primary muscle of vocal fold abduction and becomes active at the end of the normal pharyngeal phase of swallow.

During the swallow, the vocal folds (thyroarytenoids) become shorter and more massive. The cartilaginous portion of the posterior vocal folds and aryepiglottic folds adduct (transverse and oblique arytenoid muscles) to form a tight closure for safe passage of the bolus as it heads towards the upper esophageal sphincter (UES).

The Upper Esophageal Sphincter

The UES provides a high-pressure zone between the pharynx and the esophagus, remaining closed at rest, serving to separate the laryngopharynx from the esophagus. Three muscles contribute to the formation of the UES, the cricopharyngeus muscle, the most inferior muscle fibers of the inferior constrictor muscle, and the most superior portion of the longitudinal esophageal muscular fibers.[34] These three muscles attach to the posterior lamina of the cricoid cartilage. At rest, the posterior aspect of the cricoid cartilage is in contact with the posterior hypopharyngeal wall. On elevation of the larynx away from the posterior pharyngeal wall, the post-cricoid region separates from the posterior hypopharyngeal wall, thereby creating a stretching effect on the UES.[35]

The cricopharyngeus maintains normal muscle tone and relaxes during the swallow.[36] Studies have shown that UES relaxation takes place during elevation of the hyoid and larynx and reaches its most complete relaxation at maximum elevation of the hyoid/laryngeal complex.[37] At that point, the cricoid cartilage is pulled forward by the action of the hyoid bone and contraction of the thyrohyoid muscle. The UES closes, the larynx lowers, and the UES ultimately returns to its open position. There is evidence that the UES maintains contraction for a period prior to returning to its basal tone. This delay is presumed to lessen or eliminate the possibility of immediate regurgitation once the food is delivered into the esophagus.[38]

Esophageal Phase

The esophagus is a long tube that extends from the pharynx and widens as it reaches the stomach. It is generally divided into three segments, the cervical, thoracic, and abdominal segments, with the thoracic segment being the longest.[39] The cervical esophagus contains the UES, which is called the cricopharyngeus sphincter. The outer muscle fibers are arranged longitudinally, and the inner fibers area configured circularly. The propagation of the bolus, known as the peristaltic wave, actually is thought to be two waves. The first wave diminishes at the end of the cervical esophagus, and the second wave continues through the thoracic and abdominal esophagus. The thoracic esophagus begins where the striated and smooth muscles join and extends inferior to the abdominal esophagus, called the lower esophageal sphincter (LES). The LES is an anatomic sphincter.

The lower esophagus, sometimes referred to as the abdominal esophagus, contains the LES, an anatomic sphincter of circular muscles. Both the UES and LES are approximately 2 cm long; the remainder of the esophagus ranges from about 17 to 22 cm in length.

Esophageal Control

The esophageal wall is a three-layered structure consisting of the epithelium, the lamina propria, and the muscularis. The esophagus maintains its shape due to the connective tissue that lies below the epithelium in the lamina propria. The esophagus derives both afferent and efferent stimulation primarily from the vagus nerve. The muscularis layer of the esophagus contains the major neural networks that control movement of the bolus through the esophagus.[40]

The afferent paths from the esophagus travel to the central tract of the nucleus solitarius. Sensory fibers in the esophagus extend up from the LES, the esophageal body, and the UES. Sympathetic and parasympathetic paths carry impulses from the brainstem to the esophagus.[40] The paths become aligned with the enteric nerves in the submucosa of the esophagus. One set of nerves, the myenteric plexus, provides the majority of motor and secretory functions of the esophagus.

The cervical esophagus takes its innervation from the recurrent branch of CN X. The thoracic esophagus receives innervation from the recurrent branch of CN X and from the vagus nerve itself. The vagus courses downward to innervate the abdominal section of the esophagus and also sends branches to the gastrointestinal viscera. With both sensory and motor control of the esophagus by the recurrent laryngeal nerve and branches of the vagus, it is not surprising that injury or destruction to nerves in the esophagus may have implications for both swallowing and phonation.

Brainstem

The brainstem, or infratentorial, area involved in the control of swallowing is located in the dorsal region of the brainstem and adjacent to the nucleus of the tractus solitarius and in the ventral area in and around the nucleus ambiguus.[41] The brainstem is responsible for the involuntary phases of swallowing. The dorsal and ventral medullary regions in the brainstem that control swallowing have bilateral representation. Either side may control these involuntary phases. However, because of their interconnections, adequate function on both sides of the medulla is necessary for a temporally normal swallow.[42]

6. SUMMARY

The physiology of swallowing involves sensory and motor functions of the cranial nerves. Swallowing actions are both voluntary and involuntary. Although the phases of swallowing are generally thought to occur sequentially, recent evidence suggests that, in fact, the oral and oropharyngeal phases are interdependent. Martin-Harris and colleagues recently presented evidence obtained from measuring the onset times and respiratory measures associated with swallowing. Using confirmatory factor analysis, they concluded that there is an overlap between the start of the oral and pharyngeal activities of swallowing.[43] In conclusion, a thorough knowledge of swallowing physiology enhances the clinician's ability to obtain the most information from the FEESST exam. With the mechanism of the swallow understood, attention now turns to the nuts and bolts of performing the FEESST.

REFERENCES

1. Zamir Z, Ren J, Hogan W, Shaker R. Coordination of deglutitive vocal cord closure and oral-pharyngeal swallowing events in the elderly. *Eur J Gastroenterol Hepatol.* 1996;8:425–429.
2. Langmore SE, Schatz K, Olsen N. Fiberoptic endoscopic examination of swallowing safety: a new procedure. *Dysphagia.* 1988;2:216–219.
3. Bastian RW. Videoendoscopic evaluation of patients with dysphagia: an adjunct to modified barium swallow. *Otolaryngol Head Neck Surg.* 1991;104:339–350.
4. Aviv JE, Martin JH, Kim T, Sacco RL, Thomson JE, Diamond B, Close LG. Laryngopharyngeal sensory discrimination testing and the laryngeal adductor reflex. *Ann Otol Rhinol Laryngol.* 1999;108:725–730.
5. Jafari S, Prince RA, Kim DY, Paydarfar D. Sensory regulation of swallowing and airway protection: a role for the internal superior laryngeal nerve in humans. *J Physiol.* 2003;550:287–304.
6. Lee CD, Folsom AR, Blair SN. Physical activity and stroke risk: a meta-analysis. *Stroke.* 2003;34:2475–2481.
7. Ramsey DJ, Smithard DG, Kalra L. Early assessments of dysphagia and aspiration risk in acute stroke patients. *Stroke.* 2003;34:1252–1257.

8. Hilker R, Poetter C, Findeisen N, Sobesky J, Jacobs A, Neveling M, Heiss WD. Nosocomial pneumonia after acute stroke: implications for neurological intensive care medicine. *Stroke.* 2003;34:975–981.

9. Muder RR. Pneumonia in residents of long-term care facilities: epidemiology, etiology, management, and prevention. *Am J Med.* 1998; 105:319–330.

10. Marrie TJ Community-acquired pneumonia in the elderly. *Clin Infect Dis.* 2000;31:1066–1078.

11. Loeb M, McGreer A, McArthur M, Walter S, Simor AE. Risk factors for pneumonia and other lower respiratory tract infections in elderly residents of long-term care facilities. *Arch Intern Med.* 1999;159:2058–2064.

12. Siddique R, Neslusan CA, Crown WH, Crystal-Peters J, Sloan S, Farup C. A national inpatient cost estimate of percutaneous endoscopic gastrostomy (PEG)-associated aspiration pneumonia. *Am J Manag Care.* 2000; 6:490–496.

13. Niederman MS, McCombs JS, Unger AN, Kumar A, Popovian R. The cost of treating community-acquired pneumonia. *Clin Ther.* 1998;20: 820–837.

14. Kaplan V, Angus DC, Griffin MF, Clermont G, Watson RS, Linde-Zwirble WT. Hospitalized community-acquired pneumonia in the elderly: age- and sex-related patterns of care and outcome in the United States. *Am J Respir Crit Care Med.* 2002;165:766–772.

15. Marik PE, Kaplan D. Aspiration pneumonia and dysphagia in the elderly. *Chest.* 2003;124:328–336.

16. Logemann JA *Evaluation and Treatment of Swallowing Disorders.* San Diego, Calif: College-Hill Press; 1983:18–19.

17. Perlman AL. Disordered swallowing. In: Tomblin JB, Morris, HL, Spriestersbach DC, eds. *Diagnosis in Speech Language Pathology.* San Diego, Calif: Singular Publishing Group; 1994:361–383.

18. Hiiemae J, Thexton AJ, Compton AW. Intraoral food transport: the fundamental mechanism of feeding. In: Carlson DS, McNamara JA, eds. *Muscle Adaption in the Craniofacial Region.* Monograph No. 8. Ann Arbor: University of Michigan Press; 1978:181–182.

19. Kahrilas PJ, Lin S, Logemann JA, Ergun, GA, Fascchini F. Deglutive tongue action: volume accommodation and bolus propulsion. *Gastroenterology.* 1993:104:152–162.

20. Aviv JE. The normal swallow. In: Carrau, RL, Murry T, eds. *Comprehensive Management of Swallowing Disorders.* San Diego, Calif: Singular Publishing Group; 1999:23–24.

21. Pansky B, Allen DJ, Budd GC. *Review of Neurosciences.* 2nd ed. New York, NY: Macmillan Co; 1988.

22. Thexton AJ, Hiiemae KM, Crompton AW. Food consistency and bite size as regulators of jaw movement during feeding in the cat. *J Neurophysiol.* 1980;44:456–474.

23. Capra NF. Mechanics of oral sensation. *Dysphagia.* 1995;10:235–247.

24. Zemlin WR. *Speech and Hearing Science Anatomy and Physiology.* 3rd ed. Englewood Cliffs, NJ: Prentice-Hall; 1988:277.

25. Ali GN, Laundl TM, Wallace KL, deCarle, DJ, Cook, IJ. Influence of cold stimulation on the normal pharyngeal swallow response. *Dysphagia*. 1992;6;11:2–8.

26. Ludlow CL, Van Pelt F, Koda J. Characteristics of late responses to superior laryngeal nerve stimulation in humans. *Ann Otol Rhinol Laryngol*. 1992;101:127–134.

27. McConnel FMS, Cerenko D, Mendelsohn MS. Manoflourographic analysis of swallowing. *Otolaryngol Clin North Am*. 1988;21:625–635.

28. Shaker R, Dodds WJ, Danas RO, Hogan WJ, Arndorfer RC. Coordination of deglutitive glotttic closure with oropharyngeal swallowing. *Gastroenterology*. 1990;98:1478–1484.

29. Wilson JA, Pryde A, White A, Maher L, Maran AC. Swallowing performance in patients with vocal fold motion impairment. *Dysphagia*. 1995;10:149–154.

30. Mu L, Sanders I. Sensory nerve supply of the human oro- and laryngopharynx: a preliminary study. *Anat Rec*. 2000;258:406–420.

31. Olsson R, Nilsson H, Ekberg O. Simultaneous videoradiography and pharyngeal solid state manometry (videomanometry) in 25 nondysphagic volunteers. *Dysphagia*. 1995;10:36–41.

32. Ogura JH, Lam RL. Anatomical and physiological correlation on stimulating the human superior laryngeal nerve. *Laryngoscope*. 1953;63: 947–959.

33. Aviv JE, Martin JH, Keen MS, Debell M, Blitzer A. Air-pulse quantification of supraglottic and pharyngeal sensation: a new technique. *Ann Otol Rhinol Laryngol*. 1993;102:777–780.

34. Lang IM, Shaker R. Anatomy and physiology of the upper esophageal sphincter. *Am J Med*. 1997;103:50S–55S.

35. Brasseur JG, Dodds WJ. Interpretation of intraluminal manometric measurements in terms of swallowing mechanics. *Dysphagia*. 1991; 6:100–119.

36. Elidan J, Shochina M, Gonen B, Gay I. Electromyography of the inferior constrictor and cricopharyngeal muscles during swallowing. *Ann Otol Rhinol Laryngol*. 1990;99:466–469.

37. Kahrilas PJ, Dodds WJ, Dent J, Logemann JA, Shaker R. Upper esophageal sphincter opening during deglutition. *Gastroenterology*. 1988;95:52–62.

38. Kahrilas PJ. Upper esophageal sphincter function during antegrade and retrograde transit. *Am J Med*. 1997;103:56S–60S.

39. Perlman AL, Christian J. Topography and functional anatomy of the swallowing structures. In: Perlman AL, Delrieu K, eds. *Deglutition and Its Disorders*. San Diego, Calif: Singular Publishing Group; 1999:27–29.

40. Fraser C, Rothwell J, Power M, Hobson A, Thompson D, Hamdy S. Differential changes in human pharyngoesophageal motor excitability induced by swallowing, pharyngeal stimulation, and anesthesia. *Am J Physiol Gastrointest Liver Physiol*. 2003;285:G137–G144.

41. Jean A. Brainstem organization of the swallowing network. *Brain Behav Evol*. 1984;25:109–116.

42. Neumann S, Bucholz D, Jones B, Palmer J. Pharyngeal dysfunction after lateral medullary infarction is bilateral: review of 15 additional cases. [Abstract.] *Dysphagia.* 1995;10:136.
43. Martin-Harris B, Michel Y, Castell DO. Physiologic model of oropharyngeal swallowing revisited. Presented at AAO–HNS Annual Meeting; September 20, 2004; New York, NY.

II

FEESST Technique

1. Instrumentation
2. Examination of the nose, pharynx, and larynx
3. Method
4. Summary

1. INSTRUMENTATION

Introduction

The equipment necessary to perform FEESST includes a transnasal flexible laryngoscope, a sensory stimulator, a camera, a light source, a video monitor, and an analog or digital recording device (Fig 2–1). When laryngopharyngeal sensory testing was first developed in 1993, a specially designed 35-cm long transnasal flexible endoscope (called the sensory endoscope) that contained a 1.2-mm working channel (Pentax Precision Instrument Corporation, Orangeburg, NY) was used to perform sensory testing. The disadvantage of having a specially designed endoscope for sensory testing was the need for clinicians to purchase an additional flexible endoscope in order to perform the test. Another disadvantage was the inherent difficulty, and added personnel costs, of adequately cleaning, or reprocessing, a channeled endoscope. That was the state of the art until 2002, when a sensory endosheath (Vision Sciences, Natick, Mass) was developed that allowed sensory testing to be performed using almost any commercially available, 30-cm long transnasal flexible endoscope (Karl Storz Endoscopy-America, Culver City, Calif; Medtronic Xomed, Jacksonville, FL; Olympus America, Melville, NY; Pentax; Vision Sciences; Welch Allyn, Skaneateles Falls, NY). The sensory endosheath is a single-use, disposable sheath that obviates the need to use endoscope cleaning agents. The sheath is especially useful for those who examine patients in various settings such as intensive care units or at other bedside locations as it allows the examiner to do consecutive examinations without the need to carry potentially toxic endoscope cleaning agents.[1-3] Today, sensory testing can be performed using either a regular transnasal flexible laryngoscopy (TFL) scope with sensory endosheath or a sensory endoscope with the working channel without an endosheath.

The sensory stimulator is a specially designed and calibrated device that administers a discrete pulse of air that is 50 milliseconds (ms) in duration (Pentax; Vision Sciences) (Fig 2–2). The 50-ms air pulse is triggered by a foot pedal that is attached to the device. The device also contains an option to administer continuous air stimulation. It is used when no response to the 50-ms air pulse at any pressure is obtained.

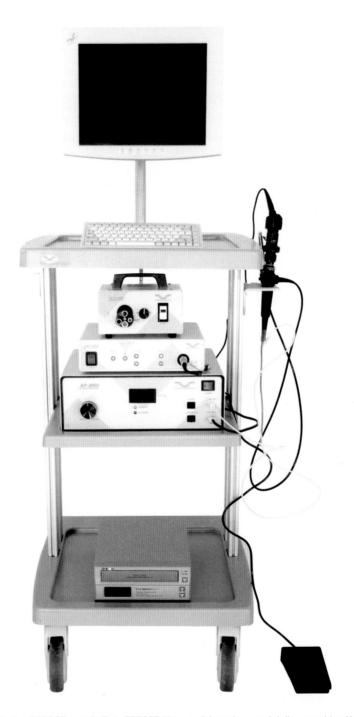

FIGURE 2-1. FEESST cart. This FEESST "tower" has top, middle, and bottom shelves. On the top shelf is the video monitor. On the middle shelf are three components: a light source sitting atop a camera, which is sitting atop the air pulse sensory stimulator. On the bottom shelf is a video recorder.

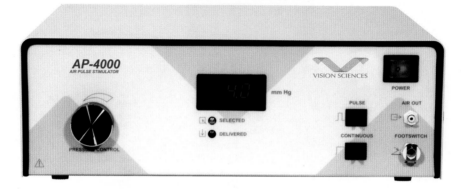

FIGURE 2–2. Air pulse sensory stimulator. Moving from left to right across the face of the device the following features are to be noted:

1. The dial, or rheostat, on the far left of the device controls the strength of the administered air pulse.
2. Digital display, in the middle of the device, which lets the clinician know what air pulse strengths are being delivered. The yellow "selected" light indicates when an air pressure is selected by turning the rheostat. The green "delivered" light appears when the foot pedal is depressed and an air pulse is administered.
3. Pulse and Continuous levers. The Pulse lever delivers a 50 ms air pulse. The Continuous lever delivers a continuous air pulse stream as long as the lever is pressed. Currently, a continuous air pulse can only be delivered by manually depressing the lever (the foot pedal only delivers 50 ms air pulses).
4. Green power switch. This power switch turns the power for the device on or off.
5. Air out. The catheter carrying the air pulse from the device to the endoscope, or to the endosheath on a scope, is attached to this portion of the air pulse device.
6. Footswitch. The foot pedal that controls the delivery of the 50 ms air pulse is attached at this portion of the air pulse device.

Calibration of the Air Pulse Sensory Stimulating Device

Correct positioning of the patient is the first step in performing a safe and patient comfortable FEESST examination. If possible, the patient should be sitting upright in an examining chair, with both hands resting gently on the knees, bending forward at the waist with the head slightly extended. This position moves the larynx away from the posterior pharyngeal wall, thereby widening the space between the laryngeal surface of the epiglottis and the posterior hypopharyngeal wall so it is easier to pass the scope toward the arytenoid to perform sensory testing.

Prior to placing the flexible endoscope into the nasal cavity, whether using the sensory endoscope (nonsheath system) or the sensory endosheath system, the sensory stimulating device must be calibrated to accommodate the ambient air pressure in the room where the sensory test is taking place.

The following steps are necessary to correctly calibrate the sensory stimulator:

1. Connect the airline from the sensory stimulator machine to the Luer lock mechanism located on sensory endoscope or on sensory endosheath (Fig 2–3).
2. Turn on sensory stimulator by depressing the green off-on power switch (see Fig 2–2).
3. Watch as the LED readout then automatically counts down 30 seconds in decreasing numbers with the display reading "C 30, C29, C28 . . . " down to C1 until the display reads "CAL".
4. When "CAL" appears on the LED display, adjust the pressure delivery dial to increase or decrease the strength of the administered air pulse until "6.0" mm Hg appears on the LED display.
5. Once 6.0 mm Hg appears, depress the foot pedal until a green light appears adjacent to the LED display. Typically, the foot pedal should be pressed twice for the green light to appear. When the green light appears, the sensory stimulator is calibrated.

While the sensory stimulator is calibrating, a small amount of surgical lubricant and defog solution is placed on the sheathed or unsheathed endoscope near the tip. The endoscope then is ready to be placed into the nasal cavity. The surgical lubricant should be kept off the tip of the endoscope or the sheath to avoid distortion or a "fogged" appearance.

When using the sensory endosheath system, the sensory endosheath has to be placed on the TFL endoscope before calibrating

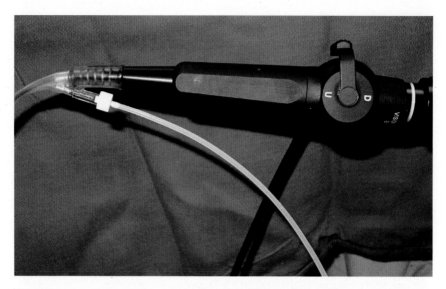

FIGURE 2–3. Luer lock of sheath on scope. The white tip of the air catheter is shown attached to the clear Luer lock located on a sensory endosheath. When not using the sensory endosheath, the white air catheter tip attaches directly to a Luer lock mechanism on the sensory endoscope.

the device. There is a particular method to correctly placing the sheath on the endoscope:

1. Orient the endoscope so that the lever that moves the scope tip is facing upward.
2. The tiny air port on the sensory endosheath *must be* directed at the 6 o'clock position on the endoscope. Therefore, it very much matters how the sensory sheath is placed on the TFL endoscope. If the lever on the endoscope is facing upward, the endosheath needs to be placed so that the catheter, which delivers the air (the "airline") from sensory stimulator machine, is 180° away from the scope lever (Fig 2–4). In this way, the air pulse is necessarily directed toward the arytenoid cartilages. Any other location of the air pulse opening will lead to imprecise air pulse administration in other regions of the hypopharynx.
3. Once the endosheath is placed on the endoscope, the clinician should visually inspect the tip of the sheathed endoscope to make sure that the air opening is indeed at the most inferior aspect of the endoscope.

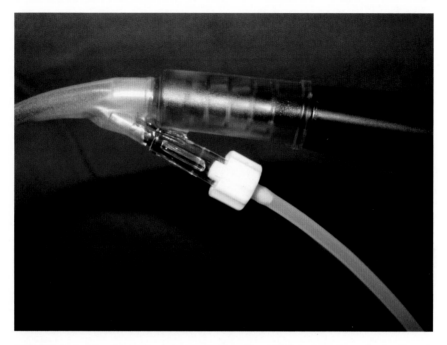

FIGURE 2–4. Placement of sensory sheath on TFL scope. In order for the air pulse to be administered inferiorly toward the arytenoid epithelium the Luer lock is located 180 degrees away from the lever of the flexible endoscope.

2. EXAMINATION OF THE NOSE, PHARYNX, AND LARYNX

Endoscopic Examination of the Nose and Pharynx

The FEESST scope is placed transnasally in the side of the nasal cavity that is most patent. Therefore, prior to endoscope placement, an examination of the nasal cavity should take place to determine the side that is less obstructed. There are two ways of transnasally passing the endoscope to ensure a quick and painless delivery into the oropharynx. The first choice is to pass it along the floor of the nose, inferior and medial to the inferior turbinate (Fig 2–5). The second choice is to pass the endoscope between the middle and inferior turbinates (Fig 2–6). Practically, this means that the scope is directed just along the inferior aspect of the middle turbinate. The nasal anatomy and the experience of the examiner will generally guide the entry of the endoscope successfully through the nasal cavity.

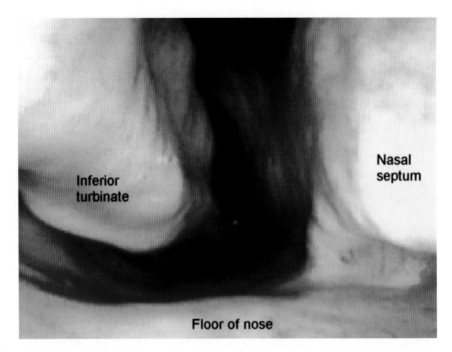

FIGURE 2-5. Right floor of nose. Endoscopic view of right nasal cavity, which shows an unobstructed right floor of nose. The floor of the nose is the first choice of where to pass the flexible laryngoscope through the nasal cavity.

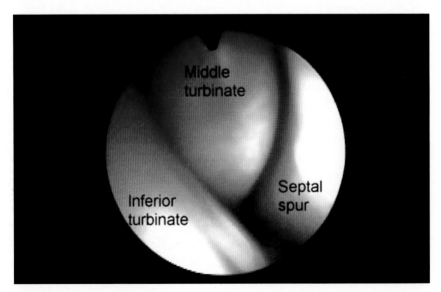

FIGURE 2-6. Right intranasal narrowing. Endoscopic view of right nasal cavity demonstrating a bone spur that is jutting into a swollen middle and inferior turbinate. When the endoscopic image shows such narrowing, it is usually prudent to pass the scope along the floor of the nose.

Since both the sensory endoscope and a standard transnasal flexible laryngoscope with sensory endosheath are quite small, about 4.3 mm in maximum diameter, it is extremely rare for the clinician to be unable to pass either scope transnasally. The most common area of intranasal narrowing is usually where a septal spur juts into the region between the middle and inferior turbinates (Fig 2–6), hence the reason the inferior-to-middle turbinate pathway of endoscope passage through the nose is the second choice. When narrowing of one side of the nasal cavity is encountered, the scope should be removed and the opposite side of the nasal cavity should be utilized because the opposite side will usually be more patent. When nasal polyps are seen (Chapter I, Fig 1–5), it is preferable to pass the scope on the side where the polyps are smallest, or to place it inferior to the location of the polyps. Variations in nasal cavity anatomy such as septal perforation and polyposis should be indicated in the medical report and a referral to a physician with expertise in rhinology suggested.

Once the scope is passed to the posterior portion of the nasal cavity, the velopharyngeal opening should be thoroughly inspected. Velopharyngeal closure can be assessed by having the patient say "kay, kay" or "cookie." A competent velopharynx will show rapid closure and release during the production of "kay." In patients with certain types of chronic neurologic disease, or after surgery or radiation therapy to the nasopharynx, the velopharynx may be incompetent (showing little or no motion during "kay" production) and can contribute to nasal air escape during a swallow. This can result in insufficient pressure buildup during propulsion of the bolus and impair the swallow. The lack of adequate closure does not necessarily indicate a swallowing disorder nor may it have anything to do with the patient's complaint. Nonetheless, if velopharyngeal incompetence is noted, it should be reported.

After the endoscope is passed through the nasopharynx, the taurus tubaris of the eustachian tubes should be inspected. On occasion, tumors in the nasopharynx can obstruct the eustachian tube opening and the patient may also complain of unilateral hearing loss. Once past the taurus, the endoscope is directed inferiorly and the base of tongue, valeculla, and supraglottic structures are visualized. A detailed endoscopic analysis of the tongue base and valeculla should take place, taking particular note of asymmetry between the right and left sides of the oropharynx and then, further inferiorly, the hypopharynx. Tumors of the tongue base, vallecula, supraglottic larynx, and lateral pharyngeal walls can be readily detected by taking the time to turn the endoscope tip right and left during this portion of the FEESST (Fig 2–7).

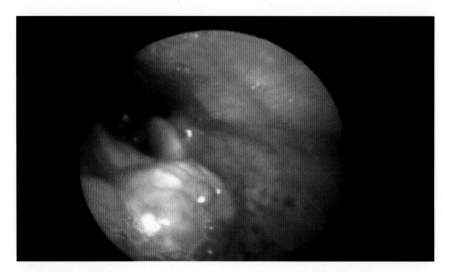

FIGURE 2–7. Base of tongue mass. Endoscopic view of tongue base and hypopharynx demonstrating a round, reddish mass protruding from the tongue base and slightly overhanging the epiglottis. This lesion turned out to be a squamous cell cancer in a patient who presented with dysphagia and had a FEESST to evaluate the dysphagia complaint.

Subsequent to the tongue base investigation, and before the larynx is examined, a "pharyngeal squeeze" maneuver should take place. The pharyngeal squeeze is a quick and simple way to assess pharyngeal motor strength by having the patient produce a 3-second high pitch "eeeeee" or the word "owl" and observing the lateral to medial excursion of the lateral pharyngeal walls.[4] When a pharyngeal squeeze is absent—that is, the pharyngeal walls do not move in response to verbal stimulation—the likelihood of concomitant laryngopharyngeal sensory deficits and laryngeal penetration and aspiration is quite high.[5,6] Furthermore, a weak or absent pharyngeal squeeze is often the first sign of an abnormal swallow.

Endoscopic Examination of the Larynx

When the larynx is examined, attention should first be focused on the presence of epithelial and subepithelial laryngeal masses and then on the symmetry of vocal fold motion. Details of endolaryngeal anatomy, especially as they pertain to acid reflux disease should be recorded (see Chapter IV). Clinically, by having the patient say a prolonged "eeee" followed immediately by a sniff, symmetry of vocal fold motion can be precisely assessed. It is for this reason, among other reasons, that the use of a video camera and recorder are extremely useful. The examiner typically wants to review the "eeee-sniff" task. If the result of the image review is asymmetry of vocal fold motion, the examiner makes recommendations for either laryngeal electromyography (EMG) or radiologic imaging of the head and neck to rule out pathology along the course of the vagus nerve. If asymmetry of vocal fold motion is observed, sensory testing should begin on the side of the larynx that appears less mobile, as the odds of even a subtle sensory deficit are higher in patients with an ipsilateral vocal fold motor problem. It is always easier to approach the arytenoid epithelium on the more numb side of the larynx.

Presence or absence of piriform sinus secretions is then noted. In addition, symmetry of the piriform sinuses is assessed. If there are copious secretions in the piriform sinuses, an effort should be made to have the patient clear these secretions, either with a cough or a swallow. It is extremely difficult to perform laryngeal sensory testing when the larynx is sitting in a pool of secretions bubbling over into the endolarynx. Therefore, taking care to clear the piriform of secretions is helpful both to obtain a valid exam and to maintain a safe examining environment for the patient. Accumulated secretions in the postcricoid region should be noted as well, as this can indicate pathology in the esophagus such as Zenker's diverticulum, vagal nerve injury, or neoplasm.

During the TFL portion of the FEESST, attention must be paid to aspiration or penetration of secretions (Fig 2–8) because this finding will immediately increase the awareness of the clinician that more severe swallowing abnormalities may be expected as the examination proceeds. Secretions entering the airway without resulting in a cough by the patient underscore the need for assessing sensory function of the larynx before commencing with food administration trials.

3. METHOD

Sensory Testing

Laryngeal sensory testing takes place by endoscopically administering discrete, calibrated 50 ms pulses of air to the arytenoid epithelium to elicit the laryngeal adductor reflex (LAR).[7] Stimulation of the epithelium innervated by the internal branch of the superior

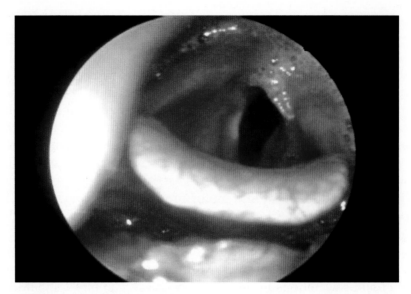

FIGURE 2–8. Aspiration of saliva. One can see the bubbles of saliva dripping from the piriform sinuses and postcricoid region onto the posterior commissure on its way to the posterior subglottic region

laryngeal nerve (SLN) elicits the LAR, which is a brief closure of the true vocal folds.[8] The LAR is an involuntary, brainstem-mediated fundamental airway protective reflex.[8,9] The sensory device delivers air pulses varying in strength from 2.0 to 10.0 mm Hg air pulse pressure. Previous work has shown that 100% of healthy controls respond to air pulse stimulation with elicitation of the LAR at air pulse strengths less than or equal to 4.0 mm Hg air pulse pressure.[10,11] Sensory discrimination thresholds are defined as normal (< 4.0 mm Hg air-pulse pressure), moderate deficits (4.0–6.0 mm Hg air-pulse pressure), or severe deficits (> 6.0 mm Hg air-pulse pressure).[10,11]

Sensory testing begins by setting the initial air pulse stimulation at a suprathreshold level of 9.0 mm Hg air pulse pressure. The reason for starting stimulation at the maximum air pulse strength is to immediately determine the patient's ability to protect his or her airway. If the patient's LAR is not elicited by the 9.0 mm Hg air pulse stimulation, the examiner has a strong indication of the patient having difficulty protecting the airway. Following a lack of response at 9 mm Hg, the examiner may now deliver *continuous* air stimulation by depressing the "continuous" lever on the sensory stimulator. At *continuous* delivery the lever is depressed for 1 second (1000 ms) to 2 seconds (2000 ms), at least 20 times as long as the typical 50 ms air pulse. If the patient's LAR is not elicited after a continuous air stream, the patient is said to have an absent LAR. Patients with an absent LAR have a statistically significant increased risk of penetrating or aspirating on any given swallow (see Chapter III). On the other hand, if the patient's LAR is elicited at 9.0 mm Hg air pulse pressure, then the air pulse strength is reduced in 1.0 mm Hg increments until the LAR is elicited. Both the right and left sides are tested.

In order to deliver the air pulse to the arytenoid epithelium, the tip of the endoscope is brought within 2 mm of the tissue surface. The foot pedal is then depressed and the air pulse delivered. The endoscopist can usually see the indentation in the tissue surface as the air pulse is delivered to the tissues. As soon as the air pulse is delivered, it is imperative for the endoscopist to withdraw the endoscope from the level of the arytenoid to a level above the epiglottis. The reason to withdraw the endoscope after stimulus delivery is that suprathreshold stimulation of the SLN not only elicits the LAR, but a swallow and cough as well. Because the larynx elevates during a swallow, a suprathreshold stimulus to the arytenoid epithelium will cause immediate laryngeal elevation; and if the endoscope is not withdrawn superiorly, an inadvertent tracheoscopy or bronchoscopy could take place.

The actual sensory discrimination threshold is then calculated by taking the mean pressure readings of the lowest pressures at which the LAR was elicited. For example, suppose the LAR is elicited on a patient at 9.0 mm Hg, 8.0 mm Hg, and 7.0 mm Hg air pulse pressure but not at 6.0 mm Hg. The reported sensory threshold is calculated as the mean between the value of the last positive pulse (7.0 mm Hg) and the last negative pulse (6.0 mm Hg), namely 6.5 mm Hg in this case. This is considered to be a severe laryngeal sensory deficit. If the clinician chooses, he or she can determine a more exact threshold by giving air pulses in 0.1 mm Hg increments and decrements between 7 and 6 mm Hg until a more precise threshold is found.

The total time needed to obtain reliable measures will vary with examiners as well as with the patient's ability to remain positioned properly (leaning forward at the waist, head in a sniffing position). Generally, sensory testing in cooperative patients rarely will take more than 5 minutes from the time the endoscope is passed into the nose until a threshold is obtained from the right and left sides of the laryngopharynx. During the sensory testing portion of the examination, attention is directed to patient management of secretions and evidence of secretions being pooled, penetrated, or aspirated is noted.

Evaluation of Swallowing

Although sensory testing may be done alone, it is usually accompanied by an examination of the patient's ability to swallow. The swallowing assessment is done after sensory testing, adhering to the philosophy of swallowing physiology, namely, airway protection first, bolus transport second. Thus, subsequent to laryngeal sensory testing, solid and liquid food of varying consistencies, dyed with green food coloring, are given to the patient. Evidence of latent swallow initiation, pharyngeal pooling and/or residue, laryngeal penetration, laryngeal aspiration and/or reflux is noted. Terminology includes:

> *Spillage:* a food bolus coursing into the hypopharynx more than 1 second before a swallowing response occurs.

> *Pharyngeal residue:* persistence of green colored material along the pharyngeal walls or within the piriform sinuses or valleculae.

> *Laryngeal penetration:* passage of material into the endolarynx but not below the vocal folds (Fig 2–9).

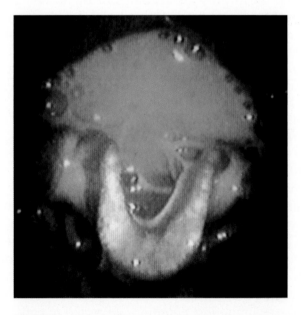

FIGURE 2–9. Laryngeal penetration. Green food material sitting in the endolarynx during a FEESST.

Aspiration: passage of material below the level of the true vocal folds into the subglottic region, trachea and bronchi.

Reflux: passage of material from the esophageal inlet retrograde into the laryngopharynx before, during, or after the
swallow.

There have been years of discussion regarding the "white-out"
period that necessarily occurs during each endoscopically observed swallow. White-out refers to the time period during a swallow where the flexible endoscope tip is momentarily blocked by
velopharyngeal closure against the posterior pharyngeal wall. The
time period of the white-out has been measured to be less than 500
ms,[12] although we have measured it to be even shorter, around 300
ms. Because most aspiration takes place before or after the swallow, the practical implications of the white-out are scant.[13] Furthermore, as soon as the white-out is over, and image motion returns to the monitor, one can readily identify green-tinged residue
below the level of the true vocal folds. If the clinician is unsure
whether or not aspiration took place at the instant of the white-out,
the bolus consistency in question can be readministered.[14] A key
point to remember here is that the images obtained during the
FEESST have to be viewed not only literally but within the context
of the general medical condition of the patient being examined. In
addition, the sensory testing information that is obtained prior to
food administration trials will also give the clinician an indication
of what to expect during the food trials. For example, as will be detailed in Chapter III, patients with a bilaterally absent LAR are at
high risk to aspirate thin liquids. Therefore, liquid administration
trials during a FEESST—after it has been determined that a patient
has severe laryngopharyngeal sensory deficits—must be given
with great caution as the patient is already known to be in a high
risk group for aspiration.

Sensory testing gives the clinician a gestalt as to what to expect
during the food administration trials. The sequence of giving solid
and liquid food consistencies is generally applied as follows:
pureed food, thickened liquid, mechanical soft food, thin liquid,
and, finally, regular food. The purpose of this sequence is to administer food consistencies that are progressively more difficult to
swallow. The solid food bolus size is altered by initially presenting
a quarter teaspoon, followed by a half teaspoon and then full teaspoon trials. Similarly, the liquid food bolus is initially presented
by spoon, then cup, and, finally, by straw. The patient is presented

with at least three repeated trials of each consistency. In an effort to simulate a typical feeding experience, patients who are capable of feeding themselves are asked to ad-lib self-administration of a meal. At times, the swallowing evaluation can take place over a 10- to 15-minute time period, further simulating a natural mealtime experience and thereby allowing the clinician to consider fatigue and its effect on swallowing function.

In some instances, the order of bolus consistency is varied. Patients may report difficulty with one or another consistency of liquid or solid food. For example, many patients with Parkinson's disease will note no difficulty with liquids but considerable difficulty with solids. In those cases, the clinician may want to start with liquids to verify the patient's report. However, the results of the sensory test are extremely important in these situations and must be considered before proceeding with the food administration trials. When a patient indicates difficulty with solids but not liquids, it may result from lack of sensory awareness of the liquid. Therefore, if the sensory test shows a severe sensory deficit, the examiner must be cautious when administering liquids as a liquid may be aspirated silently without coughing or choking by the patient.

Various compensatory and swallowing treatment strategies are attempted throughout the FEESST. Postural changes, which alter the pharyngeal dimensions or gravity's effect on bolus movement, include a chin tuck, head rotation, or a head tilt.[15,16] Therapeutic swallow maneuvers are also employed to improve airway protection, increase laryngeal elevation, and increase pharyngeal peristalsis. These maneuvers include a supraglottic swallow, a super-supraglottic swallow, an effortful swallow, and a Mendelsohn maneuver.[15,16] In addition, food viscosity and temperature are varied as well as the placement of food in the oral cavity. The purpose of these techniques is to further compensate for sensory and motor dysfunctions. By determining effective therapeutic techniques while observing the supraglottic region, intervention strategies can be employed, altered, and recorded to provide each patient with a comprehensive assessment of airway protection leading to the safest swallow possible. A safe swallow refers to a swallow that results in manageable amounts of pooling and residue and limited laryngeal penetration and aspiration.

The entire FEESST is recorded with either a digital or analog recording device. In addition, all data are recorded on a FEESST form (Fig 2–10). In this way, there are both digital and hard copy records of the FEESST evaluation. The results of the sensory and motor components of the FEESST are combined with the case his-

DATE OF EVAL m ____/d____/y____

MRN
DOB
NAME   MALE
LOCATION   FEMALE
REFERRED BY

Department of Otolaryngology / Head & Neck Surgery
Patient informed of risks, benefits & options of procedure _____

FLEXIBLE ENDOSCOPIC EVALUATION of SWALLOWING with SENSORY TESTING

Race / Ethnicity _____ (0= White / NH 1= Black 2= Hispanic 3= Asian 4=Other)
Primary Diagnosis _____
Secondary 1._____ 2._____ 3._____

HISTORY

Current Weight____lbs. Weight loss in past 3 months: (0=no 1=yes) ____ How Much?____ Height ____
Current Diet (0=no 1=yes) NPO ____ NGT ____ PEG ____ Patient able to feed self? ____
Liquid (0=honey 1=nectar 2=thin 3=none) ____ Solid (4=puree 5=mech soft 6=reg 7=none) ____
Dysphagia with (0=no 1=yes) Solids _____ Liquids _____Coughing when Eating _____ Drinking _____
History of Throat Clearing _____ Phlegm _____ Coughing _____ Heartburn/Indigestion _____
　　　　　Smoker _____ Other _____

PHYSICAL/ORAL MOTOR EXAMINATION

Smoker(0=no 1=yes) ____ Tracheotomy ____ Ventilator Dependent ____ Pretest Heart Rate(HR) _____
Lips (0=normal 1=asym 2=weak) ___ Voice Quality (0=normal 1=hoarse 2=wet 3=breathy 4=aphonic) ____
For the following (1=intact 2=impaired 3= absent)
Tongue movement ____ Tongue strength ____ Velopharyngeal competence ____ Gag ____
Volitional cough ____ Volitional swallow ____ Spontaneous swallow ____Laryngeal elevation ____

ENDOSCOPIC EXAMINATION (0=no 1=yes)

Vocal Fold Adduction Complete ____ Incomplete L /R Vocal Fold Edema____
Arytenoid Edema____ Interarytenoid/Post-com Edema ____ Erythema ____
Pharyngeal Squeeze (1=intact 2=impaired 3=absent) ____

LARYNGOPHARYNGEAL SENSORY DISCRIMINATION TEST

(+) Positive Response　　(-) Negative Response　　DATA (mmHg)
　　　　50 MSEC PULSES　　　　　　　　　CONTINUOUS AIR-PULSE DELIVERY
RIGHT _____ _____ _____ _____ 　|　　　 _____

LEFT _____ _____ _____ _____ 　|　　　 _____
　　　Normal: < 4.0 mm Hg; Moderate Deficit: 4.0-6.0 mm Hg; Severe Deficit: < 6.0 mm Hg

THRESHOLD ON LEFT _____　　　　　　THRESHOLD ON RIGHT _____

Laryngeal Sensation (0= normal 1= moderate 2= severe deficit) Right _____ Left _____
Laryngeal Adductor Response =LAR (1= right 2= left 3= bilateral) Present _____
　　　　　　　　　　　(0= LAR not elicited) Absent _____
SAFETY (0= no 1= yes) Airway Compromise _____ Epistaxis _____
Patient Rating Scale:
Comfortable (0= no 1= yes) ____ Discomfort (1=mild 2=moderate 3=severe) _____
If your physician advised you to repeat this test, would you repeat this test? (0=no 1=yes) _____

_____　　　　_____
signature of clinician　　　　　　　　**I was present for procedure**

FIGURE 2-10. FEESST Form. This is the "hard copy" of the two-page FEESST form we use at the Voice and Swallowing Center. This form can serve as the physician interpretation and report of both laryngopharyngeal sensory testing and/or FEESST. *(continues)*

Name_____ Date of Evaluation _____/_____/_____ Medical Record #_____

SWALLOWING EVALUATION

Testing Position _____ (0= chair & upright 1= chair & 45 degrees 2= bed & upright 3= bed & 45 degrees)
Pre Bolus: Pooling of Secretions (0=no 1=yes) _____   Penetration of Secretions _____
        Aspiration of Secretions   _____   Reflux of Secretions   _____

CONSISTENCIES 0=no 1=yes	Thin	Nectar	Honey	Puree	Mech Soft	Solid
Spillage						
Laryngeal Penetration						
able to clear						
Pharyngeal Residue / Pooling						
able to clear						
Aspiration						
response: silent						
cough						
able to clear						
Reflux						
able to clear						

TRIAL COMPENSATORY TECHNIQUES (0= no 1= yes)
Postural Changes _____   Other Measures _____
RISK OF ASPIRATION DUE TO (0= no 1= yes)
Poor oral control and/or copious oral residue
Diminished laryngopharyngeal sensation   _____
Premature spillage of bolus   _____
Inability to clear material from valleculae, pyriform sinus or endolarynx   _____
Reflux   _____
Post test Heart Rate (HR)   _____

IMPRESSIONS _____
_____
_____
_____
_____
_____
_____
_____

RECOMMENDATIONS
Referrals (0=no 1=yes) SLP / Dysphagia Therapy _____   GI _____   ENT:F/U _____
Diet: (0=no 1=yes)   PO _____   NPO _____   NGT _____   PEG _____
Liquid _____ (0= honey 1= nectar 2= thin 3= none)   Solid_____ (4= puree 5= mech soft 6= reg 7= none)
Position _____ (0= Chair, upright; 1= Chair , 45 degrees; 2= Bed, upright; 3= Bed, 45 degrees)
Compensatory Techniques Postural Changes____ Supervision____ (0= none 1= intermittent 2= constant)
OtherMeasures _____
_____
_____
_____
_____

_____   _____
signature of clinician   **I was present for procedure**

FIGURE 2-10. *continued.*

tory to arrive at dietary and therapeutic recommendations for the patient. The recording of the FEESST is of particular importance for several reasons. First, the results can be given to the patient's rehabilitation specialist if he or she did not perform the testing. Second, a recording of the exam allows for direct comparison during future studies. Third, without a video recording, reimbursement is not permitted. In the CPT coding system, the designation of FEESST specifically includes video recording. This is outlined in further detail in Chapter VII.

4. SUMMARY

A complete evaluation of swallowing consists of an evaluation of both airway protection and bolus transport. During the FEESST, the clinician evaluates sensory and motor functions related to the safety of swallowing. Once the examination has been completed, the clinician is able to report on the structural integrity of the swallow structures and determine to what degree it is safe for the patient to swallow and the types of foods and liquids he or she can best tolerate. The results of the examination are reported to the patient and the team members and a plan of treatment for the swallowing problem is prepared for the patient.

REFERENCES

1. Silberman HD. Non-inflatable sterile sheath for introduction of the flexible nasopharyngolaryngoscope. *Ann Otol Rhinol Laryngol.* 2001; 110:385–387.
2. Srinivasan A, Wolfenden LL, Song X, Mackie K, Hartsell TL, Jones HD, Diette GB, Orens JB, Yung RC, Ross TL, Merz W, Scheel PJ, Haponik EF, Perl TM. An outbreak of Pseudomonas aeruginosa infections associated with flexible bronchoscopes. *New Engl J Med.* 2003;348:221–227.
3. Baker KH, Chaput MP, Clavet CR, Varney GW, To TM, Lytle DC. Evaluation of endoscope sheaths as viral barriers. *Laryngoscope.* 1999; 109:636–639.
4. Bastian RW. The videoendoscopic swallowing study: an alternative and partner to the videofluoroscopic swallowing study. *Dysphagia.* 1993;8:359–367.
5. Setzen M, Cohen MA, Mattucci KF, Perlman PW, Ditkoff MK. Laryngopharyngeal sensory deficits as a predictor of aspiration. *Otolaryngol Head Neck Surg.* 2001;124,622–624.

6. Aviv JE, Spitzer J, Cohen M, Ma G, Belafsky P, Close LG. Laryngeal adductor reflex and pharyngeal squeeze as a predictor of laryngeal penetration and aspiration. *Laryngoscope.* 2002;112:338–341.

7. Aviv JE, Martin JH, Kim T, Sacco RL, Thomson JE, Diamond B, Close LG. Laryngopharyngeal sensory discrimination testing and the laryngeal adductor reflex. *Ann Otol Rhinol Laryngol.* 1999;108:725–730.

8. Ludlow CL, Van Pelt F, Koda J. Characteristics of late responses to superior laryngeal nerve stimulation in humans. *Ann Otol Rhinol Laryngol.* 1992;101:127–134.

9. Jafari S, Prince RA, Kim DY, Paydarfar D. Sensory regulation of swallowing and airway protection: a role for the internal superior laryngeal nerve in humans. *J Physiol.* 2003;550:287–304.

10. Aviv JE, Martin JH, Jones ME, Wee TA, Diamond B, Keen MS, Blitzer A. Age-related changes in pharyngeal and supraglottic sensation. *Ann Otol Rhinol Laryngol.* 1994;103:749–752.

11. Aviv JE, Martin JH, Sacco RL, Diamond B, Zagar D, Diamond B, Keen MS, Blitzer A. Supraglottic and pharyngeal sensory abnormalities in stroke patients with dysphagia. *Ann Otol Rhinol Laryngol.* 1996;105:92–97.

12. Perlman A, Van Deale D. Simultaneous videoendoscopic and ultrasound measures of swallowing. *J Med Speech Lang Pathol.* 1993;1:223–232.

13. Colodny N. Effects of age, gender, disease and multisystem involvement on oxygen saturation levels in dysphagic persons. *Dysphagia.* 2001;16:48–57.

14. Langmore SE. Evaluation of oropharyngeal dysphagia: which diagnostic tool is superior. *Curr Opin Otolaryngol Head Neck Surg.* 2003; 11:485–489.

15. Murry, T. Therapeutic intervention for swallowing disorders. In: Carrau RL, Murry T, eds. *Comprehensive Management of Swallowing Disorders.* San Diego, Calif: Singular Publishing Group; 1999:243–248.

16. Logeman, JA. Therapy for oropharyngeal swallowing disorders. In: Perlman AL, Schultz-Delrieu K, eds. *Deglutition and Its Disorders.* San Diego, Calif: Singular Publishing Group; 1997:449–462.

III

FEESST Applications and Outcomes

1. Laryngeal sensory testing in the elderly
2. Laryngeal sensory testing in stroke patients with dysphagia
3. Using FEESST to predict laryngeal penetration and aspiration
4. Outcomes: FEESST versus modified barium swallow (MBS)
5. Summary

INTRODUCTION

In this chapter, the use of FEESST in various populations is discussed. For each population, a case synopsis is given. It should be remembered that, although the FEESST is administered in the same manner as described in Chapter II, variations in test format may be required depending on the patient's ability to tolerate the test and the patient's level of cooperation. For example, it may be necessary for the examiner to have someone assist with maintaining the patient's head in a stable posture. It may also be necessary to change the order of consistencies to be swallowed. Finally, there may be some patients for whom the FEESST alone does not allow the examiner to reach a definitive decision on the dysphagia diagnosis (see the algorithm in Chapter V).

1. LARYNGEAL SENSORY TESTING IN THE ELDERLY

As people get older dysphagia and aspiration are more likely to occur.[1,2] Dysphagia in the elderly population may stem from a myriad of conditions. As one ages, minor neurologic events such as small periventricular infarcts not often visible on MRI may occur. Other factors, such as cognitive disintegration, the use of multiple medications, and the simple act of often having to eat alone, all contribute to dysphagia in the elderly.

The primary reasons for increased dysphagia in the elderly have often been ascribed to motor dysfunctions of the oral cavity and pharynx, such as lip seal difficulty, tongue fasciculations, impairment of tongue mobility, poor lingual-palatal seal, impaired pharyngeal peristalsis, and inability to close the airway during bolus passage.[3] However, the explanation is not all ascribable to motor pathology. Studies have shown that sensory dysfunction of the oral cavity takes place as well, with oral cavity sensory discriminatory ability diminishing with advancing age.[4,5] Over the past decade, it has been repeatedly demonstrated that laryngeal sensory capacity also diminishes with increasing age.[6-8] This is not surprising in that sensory functions related to taste, smell, and hearing also decrease as one ages. Thus, the sensory as well as the motor branches of the cranial nerves are subject to decreasing responsivity with aging.

A study of laryngeal sensory testing was conducted in healthy adults with no complaints of swallowing ranging in age from 23 to 87 years old, using calibrated air pulses to obtain a response. A progressive increase in sensory discrimination threshold with each decade of life was found. A correlation analysis revealed significant increases in air pulse pressure thresholds with advancing age.[6] Specifically, for people from 20 to 40 years of age, the average laryngeal sensory threshold was 2.07 mm Hg air pulse pressure; for the 41 to 60 age group, 2.22 mm Hg air pulse pressure, and for people 61 and older, 2.68 mm Hg air pulse pressure. Thresholds for the 61 and older group were significantly higher than those for both the 20 to 40 and the 41 to 60 groups.[6]

The contention that the demonstrated age-related increase in sensory discrimination thresholds may have a role in the development of dysphagia and aspiration in the elderly is supported from a landmark study of cadaveric superior laryngeal nerves.[9] The ultrastructural changes that occur with increasing age in the human superior laryngeal nerve (SLN) were examined by Mortelliti and his colleagues, who found an extensive and statistically significant decrease in the number of sensory nerve fibers in subjects over 60 years of age.[9] The aforementioned studies in both the clinical and basic science realms strongly point to airway protective capacity diminishing concomitant with the aging process. These studies suggest that clinicians should turn their attention to addressing sensory deficits as part of the treatment planning process for the elderly with dysphagia. The following clinical vignette illustrates how these basic scientific findings relate to a real-life situation.

Case Example: Sensory Testing in the Elderly

An 84-year-old female, living alone, presents with a complaint of 6 months of coughing when drinking water. She reports no weight loss or recent history of antibiotic treatment for upper respiratory infection. The patient also reports brushing her teeth once a day. The patient has a history of hypothyroidism and gastroesophageal reflux disease but is otherwise healthy—no stroke, heart attack, diabetes, or history of respiratory disorders. The patient's medications at the time of the evaluation were synthyroid, a proton pump inhibitor, and baby aspirin. A recent upper GI endoscopy on antacids revealed a moderate hiatal hernia and no other pathology. A FEESST was performed, which showed moderate laryngopharyngeal sensory deficits bilaterally at 5.5 mm Hg air pulse pressure. The laryngeal ex-

> am was unremarkable, with minimal posterior laryngeal edema, no paradoxical vocal fold motion, and good vocal fold motion on the "eee-sniff" task. During the food administration trials, there was intermittent, slight penetration of thin liquids without aspiration. Thickening the liquid to nectar and honey consistencies resulted in no penetration.

The FEESST team reviewed the exam with the patient, taking particular care to point out to her two key findings: one, that she was a bit numb in the "throat," and two, that when she drank liquids with a waterlike consistency, she occasionally had the material enter the "area close to the vocal cords." Her treatment plan was to avoid thin liquids, to thicken the liquids she will be taking, and to practice good oral hygiene—increasing the frequency of tooth brushing to three times a day. Our interpretation of this study was that the patient's intermittent cough resulted from periodic penetration of liquid material into the endolarynx likely from age-related diminution of her airway protective capacity. Diet alteration and improved oral hygiene provided a straightforward, low morbidity means of addressing this subtle physiologic problem of laryngopharyngeal hyposensitivity. On her return visit 10 weeks later, she noted improved swallowing with almost total elimination of the cough after drinking liquids that were slightly thickened.

2. LARYNGEAL SENSORY TESTING IN STROKE PATIENTS WITH DYSPHAGIA

Cerebral vascular accidents (CVAs) are not only devastating because of swallowing disorders; when severe, they often require significant rehabilitative efforts from all members of the rehabilitation team. After a CVA, patients may exhibit reluctance to swallowing and cognitive deficits that result in oral containment, drooling, facial weakness, and oral apraxias. These issues may confound the assessment of swallow safety, thus requiring the work of the entire dysphagia team to manage the patient's rehabilitation. This section is not intended to describe the pathophysiology of CVAs; however, when attempting to manage a patient after a CVA, it should be remembered that the type of stroke (ie, brainstem or infratentorial, and cortical or supratentorial) might have certain clinical features and the rehabilitation team must remain aware of the underlying pathophysiology. Critical in the patient's recovery is the awareness of both motor and sensory control of the act of swallowing.

After a stroke, patients are at high risk for developing aspiration pneumonia. Choking on foods or liquids may also cause them to reduce food intake to a level that is below their nutritional needs. Several studies have examined the sensory and motor abilities of individuals following strokes.

To determine if stroke patients with dysphagia have laryngopharyngeal sensory deficits, laryngeal sensory thresholds were prospectively assessed in a cohort with supratentorial (cortical) and/or infratentorial (brainstem) stroke. Age-matched controls were sensory tested as well.[10] No sensory deficits were found in any of the age-matched controls. However, in all stroke patients studied, either unilateral or bilateral laryngeal sensory deficits were identified. Statistically, these mean elevations (left and right sides averaged) in sensory discrimination thresholds were significantly greater than the thresholds of age-matched controls. Among patients with unilateral sensory deficits, sensory thresholds were significantly elevated in all cases on the affected side compared with the unaffected side. Moreover, the sensory thresholds of the unaffected side were not significantly different from those of the age-matched controls.[10]

The results of this study demonstrated that stroke patients with dysphagia have sensory deficits in the laryngopharynx and underscore the fact that problems with laryngopharyngeal sensation should be addressed in the diagnosis and management of stroke patients with dysphagia.

Case Example: Sensory Testing in Stroke Patient

A 66-year-old male was hospitalized as a result of a right brainstem stroke. The patient complained of difficulty swallowing solid foods and liquids, and a FEESST was ordered. The FEESST revealed a severe sensory deficit on the right, and normal sensory thresholds on the left.

This sensory information guided the swallowing team to have the patient turn his head to the right—toward the numb side of the hypopharynx—during a swallow so the numb portion of the hypopharynx would be effectively narrowed, thereby allowing an incoming food bolus to be redirected toward the left, or more sensate, side of the pharynx. Endoscopic observation of this swallow maneuver demonstrated improved swallow with no penetration or aspiration of food or thickened liquids. The patient's diet and positioning during mealtime (head turn) was modified with satisfaction.

3. USING FEESST TO PREDICT LARYNGEAL PENETRATION AND ASPIRATION

The previous section demonstrated that FEESST can be utilized to precisely guide dietary and behavioral management of stroke patients with swallowing problems. This section will show that FEESST has an essential, broad role in dysphagia management, regardless of the etiology of the dysphagia.

FEESST was prospectively studied in 133 adult patients with dysphagia who had a variety of underlying diagnoses, with stroke and chronic neurologic disease—Parkinson's disease, bulbar palsy, multiple sclerosis, amyotrophic lateral sclerosis, pseudobulbar palsy—predominating.[11] In 75% of the patients studied, unilateral or bilateral severe laryngopharyngeal sensory deficits were found. Almost half of the patients with severe laryngopharyngeal deficits, compared to less than 10% of patients with either normal sensation or moderate sensory deficits, displayed aspiration. This study was the first to suggest an association between sensory deficits and the development of laryngeal penetration or aspiration on any given swallow.

To further delineate the contribution of laryngopharyngeal sensory deficits to the outcome of a swallow and to establish the relationship between sensory and motor deficits in the laryngopharynx, another prospective study was performed.[12] The purpose of the study was to determine if patients with laryngopharyngeal sensory and motor deficits were at increased risk for laryngeal penetration and aspiration during swallowing and to determine the relationship between pharyngeal motor weakness and laryngeal sensory deficits. FEESST was performed on 122 patients with dysphagia who were prospectively divided into two groups. The control group consisted of 76 patients with normal laryngeal sensory thresholds (LAR elicited at <4.0 mm Hg air pulse pressure), and the study group consisted of 46 patients with an absent LAR (no LAR elicited after *continuous* air pulse stimulation). Each patient in each group was given a teaspoon of pureed food, followed by a teaspoon of thin liquid. The presence or absence of laryngeal penetration and aspiration was recorded. Pharyngeal muscle strength was assessed by noting presence or absence of the pharyngeal squeeze, elicited by having the patient produce a high-pitched "eeee" sound.

The results of the swallowing portion of the study are detailed in Figure 3–1. The patients with an absent LAR, when taking thin liquids, had a 100% risk of laryngeal penetration and a 94% risk of aspiration. These findings were significantly higher than the control group of dysphagic patients with normal LARs. Similar findings were noted with puree consistencies, that is, the absent LAR group had a significantly higher risk of penetration and aspiration compared with the patients with normal airway protective reflexes.

When incorporating pharyngeal squeeze data, the following was shown: In controls (normal LAR) with dysphagia, pharyngeal squeeze was impaired in only about 20% with a small incidence of penetration and aspiration. In contrast, in the absent LAR group, pharyngeal squeeze—the motor side of pharyngeal function—was impaired in almost 90% of patients, with penetration occurring in 95% and aspiration in nearly 80%. The difference in the prevalence of pharyngeal weakness between the normal LAR and absent LAR groups was significant. The difference in the prevalence of penetration and aspiration was significantly higher in the absent LAR/impaired pharyngeal contraction cohort than in the normal sensation/impaired contraction cohort. Other investigators have shown similar findings.[13,14]

The studies reported above support the contention that the absence of the LAR and impaired pharyngeal squeeze puts patients with dysphagia at high risk for laryngeal penetration and aspiration compared to patients with an intact LAR and intact pharyngeal squeeze. Moreover, these findings suggest a strong association between motor and sensory deficits in the laryngopharynx.

Because of these findings, a **dysphagia treatment algorithm** has been developed (Fig 3–2). The essence of the algorithm is that the clinician does not have to actually see aspiration during a FEESST to be concerned that the patient is at risk for aspirating on any given swallow. If a patient with an absent LAR displays penetration during the FEESST evaluation, he or she will likely aspirate and should be given a non-oral route of alimentation. On the other hand, a patient with an intact LAR who is found to be aspirating, as long as he or she is not silently aspirating (material in the trachea and no reaction [cough, choking] by the patient), likely can be given alimentation by mouth.

When the skeptical clinician asks, "What use is sensory testing?" the answer lies in the aforementioned studies. Both MBS and

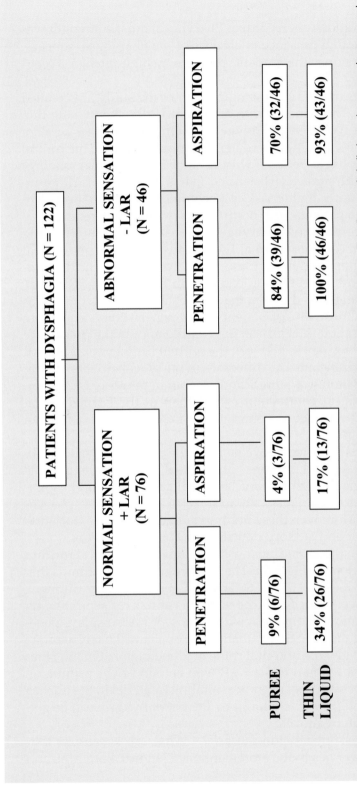

FIGURE 3–1. Laryngopharyngeal sensation, laryngeal penetration, and aspiration. This figure details how laryngopharyngeal sensory testing can predict the relative likelihood of laryngeal penetration and aspiration on any given swallow of either a puree or a thin liquid. For example, if a patient has an absent LAR, for all intents and purposes, the patient will experience laryngeal penetration when trying to drink a thin liquid. On the other hand, if the patient has an intact LAR, the likelihood of experiencing laryngeal penetration of a thin liquid is only about one-third of the time.

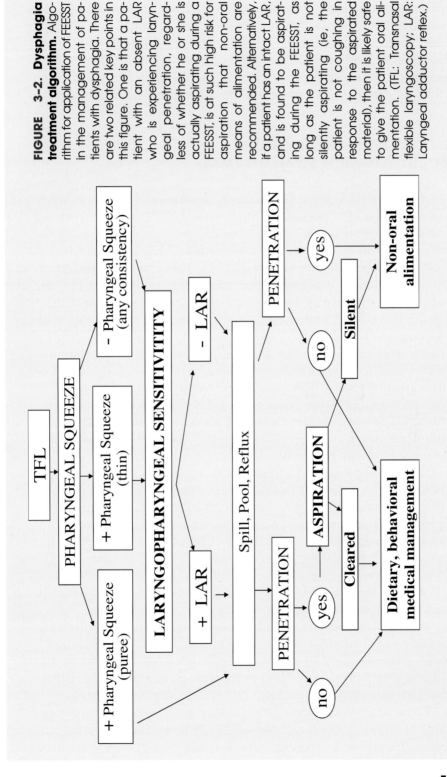

FIGURE 3–2. Dysphagia treatment algorithm. Algorithm for application of FEESST in the management of patients with dysphagia. There are two related key points in this figure. One is that a patient with an absent LAR who is experiencing laryngeal penetration, regardless of whether he or she is actually aspirating during a FEESST, is at such high risk for aspiration that non-oral means of alimentation are recommended. Alternatively, if a patient has an intact LAR, and is found to be aspirating during the FEESST, as long as the patient is not silently aspirating (ie, the patient is not coughing in response to the aspirated material), then it is likely safe to give the patient oral alimentation. (TFL: Transnasal flexible laryngoscopy; LAR: Laryngeal adductor reflex.)

FEES essentially leave the clinician with a high level of risky guess-work as to how to manage patients who are "slightly penetrating" and "slightly aspirating." The sensory testing information gives the clinician a real-time view of the patient's overall ability to protect his or her airway; hence, the true significance of a bit of penetration and aspiration can be put into immediate perspective.

4. OUTCOMES: FEESST VERSUS MODIFIED BARIUM SWALLOW (MBS)

There has never been a prospective, randomized outcome study examining the effectiveness of FEES versus MBS, or FEES versus a bedside swallowing evaluation, or MBS versus a bedside swallowing evaluation, but there has been one for FEESST versus MBS. A randomized, prospective cohort outcome study in a hospital-based outpatient setting was performed to investigate whether FEESST or MBS was superior as the diagnostic test for evaluating and guiding the behavioral and dietary management of outpatients with dysphagia.[15] One hundred and twenty-six outpatients with dysphagia were randomized to either FEESST or MBS as the diagnostic test used to guide dietary and behavioral (postural changes or alterations of food volumes and consistencies) management. The outcome variables were pneumonia incidence and pneumonia-free interval. The patients were enrolled for 1 year and followed for 1 year. There were a variety of underlying diagnoses that led to the dysphagia consultation with stroke predominating.

Seventy-eight MBS examinations were performed in 76 patients, with 14 patients (18.4%) developing pneumonia. Sixty-one FEESST examinations were performed in 50 patients, with 6 patients (12.0%) developing pneumonia. These differences were not statistically significant ($\chi^2 = 0.93$, $p = 0.33$). In the MBS group, the median pneumonia-free interval was 47 days; in the FEESST group, the median pneumonia-free interval was 39 days. Based on a Wilcoxon signed-rank test, this difference was not statistically significant ($z = 0.04$, $p = 0.96$).

In specifically examining the patients who had an underlying diagnosis of stroke, the following was noted: in the MBS group, 7 of 24 patients developed pneumonia (29.2%); whereas in the FEESST group, 1 of 21 (4.76%) developed pneumonia. This difference was statistically significant ($p = 0.05$, Fisher's exact test).

There are two reasons why dietary and behavioral management of stroke patients guided by FEESST resulted in better outcomes than those in patients whose management was guided by

MBS. One relates to the greater amount of time allowed for a FEESST compared to an MBS, so that patient fatigue and its sequelae are more readily identified and managed. Patients with stroke have been shown to experience fatigue of the pharyngeal phase of swallowing as they progress through a meal.[16,17] The other reason for the difference in stroke patient outcomes may be that information regarding the sensory component of the swallow is precisely assessed with FEESST but only indirectly addressed with MBS. As a result, the clinician using FEESST has a heightened awareness of aspiration risks that might otherwise have been overlooked.

Whether dysphagic outpatients have their dietary and behavioral management guided by the results of MBS or FEESST, their outcomes with respect to pneumonia incidence and pneumonia-free interval are essentially the same. What this means practically for the clinician and the patient is that the clinician can offer the patient an office-based test of swallowing, without the need for a radiologic facility and its attendant X-ray exposure, that can comprehensively assess the nature of the swallowing problem the patient is experiencing.

5. SUMMARY

Laryngopharyngeal sensory thresholds diminish with age and can be significantly abnormal in patients who have suffered a stroke or who have chronic neurodegenerative diseases. We believe that laryngopharyngeal sensory deficits contribute to the swallowing difficulties seen in these groups of patients. Furthermore, assessment of laryngopharyngeal sensation can be utilized to predict likelihood of laryngeal penetration and aspiration on any given swallow. Specifically, patients with severe laryngopharyngeal sensory deficits, especially those with an absent LAR, are at significantly higher risk for laryngeal penetration and aspiration compared with patients with normal laryngopharyngeal sensation. This information is critical in deciding when, and what, to feed a patient with dysphagia.

REFERENCES

1. Feinberg MJ, Ekberg O. Videofluoroscopy in elderly patients with aspiration: importance of evaluating both oral and pharyngeal stages of deglutition. *Amer J Radiol.* 1991;156:293–296.

2. Marrie TJ. Community-acquired pneumonia in the elderly. *Clin Infect Dis.* 2000;31:1066–1078.

3. Feinberg MJ, Knebl J, Tully J. Prandial aspiration and pneumonia in an elderly population followed over 3 years. *Dysphagia.* 1996;11:104–109.

4. Aviv JE, Hecht C, Weinberg H, Dalton JF, Urken ML. Surface sensibility of the floor of mouth and tongue in healthy controls and radiated patients. *Otolaryngol Head Neck Surg.* 1992;107:418–423.

5. Calhoun KH, Gibson B, Hartley L, Minton J, Hokanson JA. Age-related changes in oral sensation. *Laryngoscope.* 1992;102:109–116.

6. Aviv JE, Martin JH, Jones ME, Wee TA, Diamond B, Keen MS, Blitzer A. Age related changes in pharyngeal and supraglottic sensation. *Ann Otol Rhinol Laryngol.* 1994;103:749–752.

7. Aviv JE. Effects of aging on sensitivity of the pharyngeal and supraglottic areas. *Am J Med.* 1997;103(5A):74S–76S.

8. Aviv JE. Sensory discrimination in the larynx and hypopharynx. *Otolaryngol Head Neck Surg.* 1997;116:331–334.

9. Mortelliti AJ, Malmgren LT, Gacek RR. Ultrastructural changes with age in the human superior laryngeal nerve. *Arch Otolaryngol Head Neck Surg.* 1990;116:1062–1068.

10. Aviv JE, Martin JH, Sacco RL, Zagar D, Garber M, Huang W, Keen MS, Blitzer A. Supraglottic and pharyngeal sensory abnormalities in stroke patients with dysphagia. *Ann Otol Rhinol Laryngol.* 1996;105:92–97.

11. Aviv JE, Kim T, Goodhart K, Kaplan S, Thomson J, Diamond B, Close LG. FEESST: a new bedside endoscopic test of the motor and sensory components of swallowing. *Ann Otol Rhinol Laryngol.* 1998;107:378–387.

12. Aviv JE, Spitzer J, Cohen M, Ma G, Belafsky P, Close LG. Laryngeal adductor reflex and pharyngeal squeeze as predictors of laryngeal penetration and aspiration. *Laryngoscope.* 2002;112:338–341.

13. Perlman PW, Cohen MA, Setzen M, Baleafsky PC, Guss J, Mattucci KF, Ditkoff M. The risk of aspiration of pureed food as determined by flexible endoscopic evaluation of swallowing with sensory testing. *Otolaryngol Head Neck Surg.* 2004;130:80–83.

14. Setzen M, Cohen MA, Perlman PW, Belafsky PC, Guss J, Mattucci KF, Ditkoff M. The association between laryngopharyngeal sensory deficits, pharyngeal motor function, and the prevalence of aspiration with thin liquids. *Otolaryngol Head Neck Surg.* 2003;128:99–102.

15. Aviv JE. Prospective, randomized outcome study of endoscopy versus modified barium swallow in patients with dysphagia. *Laryngoscope.* 2000;110:563–574.

16. Hamdy S, Aziz Q, Rothwell JC, Crone R, Hughes D, Tallis RC, Thompson DG. Explaining oropharyngeal dysphagia after unilateral hemispheric stroke. *Lancet.* 1997;350:686–692.

17. Hamdy S, Aziz Q, Rothwell JC, Singh KD, Barlow J, Hughes DG, Tallis RC, Thompson DG. The cortical topography of human swallowing musculature in health and disease. *Nature Med.* 1996;11:1217–1224.

IV

Sensory Testing Alone

1. SITE OF LESION TESTING

Introduction

When a new patient comes into the physician's office complaining of hoarseness, throat clearing, increased phlegm, and cough, the standard workup of these complaints invariably involves a trans-nasal flexible laryngoscopy (TFL). The TFL, especially when combined with either an add-on camera or a distal-chip camera, can give the clinician examining the patient a precise assessment of laryngeal motor function. In addition, the camera with its accompanying recording device allows a permanent record to be made for comparison following treatments and for patient education. What video laryngoscopy cannot give the clinician is a precise assessment of laryngeal sensory function. Superior laryngeal nerve (SLN) pathology, including neuralgia, paresis, and other types of SLN dysfunction, is often a very difficult diagnosis to ascertain. The functional and anatomic integrity of the SLN, particularly its sensory, internal branch, is a critical piece of information for the physician in the investigation of common laryngopharyngeal complaints. Laryngopharyngeal sensory testing, applied as a separate test without a complete assessment of swallowing (FEESST), permits the full evaluation of laryngopharyngeal sensory function. Sensory testing, therefore, when added to standard TFL, can be considered a comprehensive test of the neurologic integrity of the larynx.

Asymmetric Laryngopharyngeal Sensory Thresholds

Because sensory testing assesses the integrity of the internal branch of the SLN, sensory deficits provide an indication of derangement of SLN function. The clinician must determine whether the problem with the SLN is a central (central nervous system) deficit or a peripheral deficit. The presence or absence of a symmetric response to laryngopharyngeal sensory testing is the first place to resolve the central deficit versus peripheral deficit question. An asymmetric response to sensory testing means that one side of the laryngopharynx has normal or near normal sensory threshold and the other side has a severe sensory deficit. The worst case would be an absent laryngeal adductor reflex (LAR). Asymmetric sensory testing findings should alert the clinician performing the test that this result may indicate a mass pressing on the vagus nerve somewhere along its route from the brainstem to skull base to neck (see Chapter

VIII, Cases). In addition, asymmetric sensory findings may indicate other central pathology such as a focal area of ischemia in the brain, a finding in certain patients with a reported transient ischemic attack (TIA).

Another cause of asymmetric laryngopharyngeal sensory thresholds occurs in patients with dysphagia, globus, and throat clearing symptoms after thyroid and parathyroid surgery. Asymmetric sensory testing findings in this setting generally indicate some type of trauma to the SLN that took place during thyroid and/or parathyroid surgery. Although laryngeal electromyography (EMG) can be helpful in assessing the integrity of the motor, or external, branch of the SLN (to the cricothyroid muscle), the sensory branch of the SLN is not assessed with laryngeal EMG. Therefore, laryngopharyngeal sensory testing can provide an immediate assessment of the internal (sensory) branch of the SLN without subjecting the patient to transcutaneous placement of fine-gauge needles through the neck.

Symmetric Laryngopharyngeal Sensory Thresholds

When the sensory thresholds are symmetric, but severely abnormal, one must consider a central etiology such as upper motor neuron disease or other chronic neurodegenerative diseases. In such cases, the severe laryngopharyngeal sensory deficits are generally not the only findings during the physical examination. One of the most important areas to examine in the head and neck of a patient who comes into the office complaining of dysphagia, globus sensation (lump in the throat), throat clearing, and hoarseness is the tongue surface. In particular, looking for tongue fasciculations may be pivotal in trying to determine the reason for the patient's symptoms. Amyotrophic lateral sclerosis (ALS) is an uncommon disease with onset in the fifth or sixth decade of life and with a male predominance. The otolaryngologist and speech-language pathologist are often the first to suspect the problem when doing an oral-motor examination of the lips, tongue, and soft palate. Sensory testing showing bilateral, severe symmetric sensory deficits along with tongue fasciculations and progressive painless weakness are hallmark signs of this disorder. Other central disorders that are likely to show bilateral sensory deficits are inflammatory myopathies and myasthenia gravis.

Tongue fasciculations, impaired tongue mobility, and impaired tongue strength in concert with symmetric, severe sensory deficits strongly suggest central neurologic pathology such as that seen with ALS, bulbar palsy, and other chronic neurologic diseases. In such cases, a referral for a complete neurologic evaluation is indicated. Thus, laryngopharyngeal sensory testing provides a valid and reliable tool for the early detection of central versus peripheral neurologic disease.

2. ACID REFLUX DISEASE

Introduction

In an otherwise healthy individual complaining of hoarseness, dysphagia, throat clearing, increased phlegm and cough, who has symmetric laryngopharyngeal sensory deficits and no additional muscle weakness, the etiology of the patient complaint is typically acid reflux injury to the laryngopharyngeal epithelium. Reflux of acid into the hypopharynx, or laryngopharyngeal reflux (LPR), is a very common and potentially debilitating chronic disease process.[1] The symptoms of LPR include hoarseness, dysphagia, globus sensation, chronic cough, and frequent throat clearing.[2,3]

Assessment of Reflux Severity

The most common symptoms of LPR have been quantified systematically by Belafsky et al.[4] From a list of common symptoms, they developed the Reflux Symptom Index (RSI, Table 4–1), a patient self-assessment questionnaire of the severity of common symptoms of reflux. An RSI of greater than 10 is significant and strongly suggests LPR. Every patient who comes into the Voice and Swallowing Center at the Columbia University Medical Center completes the RSI on his or her first visit and at all follow-up visits so that progression or regression of patient complaints can be followed. Heartburn and regurgitation, the classic symptoms of gastroesophageal reflux disease (GERD), are unusual symptoms in patients with LPR, occurring in as few as 10% of patients with LPR symptoms.[5] Although the reasons for this are not completely understood, most investigators suspect that it relates to the lack of acid clearing mechanisms in the larygopharynx.

The physical exam findings of LPR, as seen on TFL, have also been quantified by Belafsky et al, and are referred to as the Reflux Finding Score (RFS, Table 4–2).[6] The RFS is determined by a clini-

Table 4–1. Reflux Symptom Index (RSI). A score of greater than 10 strongly suggests that the patient has laryngopharyngeal reflux.

Within the last MONTH, how did the following problems affect you? (0 = no problem; 5 = severe problem):						
1. Hoarseness or problem with voice	0	1	2	3	4	5
2. Clearing your throat	0	1	2	3	4	5
3. Excess throat mucus or postnasal drip	0	1	2	3	4	5
4. Difficulty swallowing food, liquids, or pills	0	1	2	3	4	5
5. Coughing after you ate or after lying down	0	1	2	3	4	5
6. Breathing difficulties or choking episodes	0	1	2	3	4	5
7. Troublesome or annoying cough	0	1	2	3	4	5
8. Something sticking in throat or lump in throat	0	1	2	3	4	5
9. Heartburn, chest pain, indigestion	0	1	2	3	4	5

Table 4–2. Reflux Finding Score (RFS). A score of greater than 5 strongly suggests laryngopharyngeal reflux disease.

FINDINGS		SCORING		
Subglottic edema (pseudosulcus vocalis)		2 if present		
Ventricular obliteration		2 if partial		4 if complete
Erythema/hyperemia		2 arytenoids only		4 if diffuse
Vocal fold edema	1 Mild	2 Mod	3 Severe	4 Polyp
Arytenoid/ interarytenoid edema	1 Mild	2 Mod	3 Severe	4 Obstruction
Posterior commissure hypertrophy	1 Mild	2 Mod	3 Severe	4 Obstruction
Granuloma/ granulation		2 if present		
Thick endolaryngeal mucus		2 if present		

cian after the TFL and before food is given if a full FEESST examination is planned. An RFS of greater than 5 is significant and strongly suggests LPR.[6] Again, every patient being evaluated in our Voice and Swallowing Center has the RFS completed by one or both clinicians as a means of following the laryngopharyngeal signs in a patient with LPR symptoms. The RFS is a clinician-based score of eight parameters observed during TFL. Of the eight parameters, five refer to the ways in which edema of the larynx is observed. The five "edema" findings are as follows:

1. *Pseudosulcus vocalis*—refers to subglottic edema that extends from anterior to posterior all the way to the posterior commissure (Fig 4–1, Fig 4–2), thereby differentiating itself from a true sulcus vertegure, which terminates at the vocal process of the arytenoids.
2. *Ventricle obliteration*—Normally the 2 to 3 mm ventricular space between the true vocal folds and false vocal folds is apparent

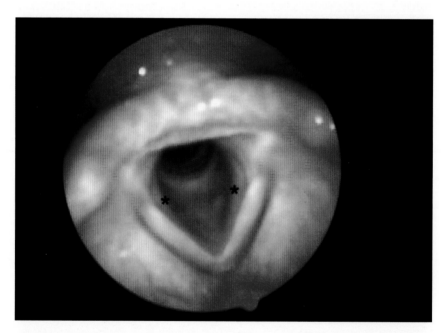

FIGURE 4–1. Pseudosulcus vocalis. Note the bilateral, subglottic edema that extends from the anterior commissure to the posterior commissure (*black asterisks*), appearing almost as a duplicate of the true vocal folds. A true sulcus vergeture terminates at the vocal process of the arytenoids, thereby differentiating itself from a pseudosulcus.

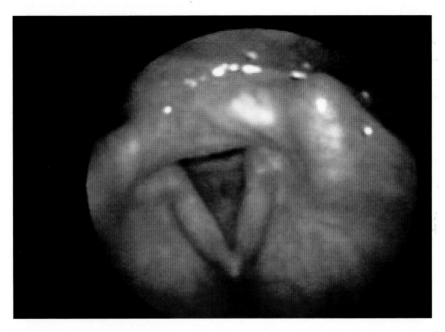

FIGURE 4–2. No pseudosulcus. Endoscopic view of the hypopharynx in a healthy control demonstrating true vocal folds without pseudosulcus vocalis.

(Fig 4–3). However, with LPR this space is obliterated (Fig 4–4).

3. *Vocal fold edema*—the true vocal folds themselves can undergo polypoid degeneration as a result of acid injury (Fig 4–4).
4. *Diffuse laryngeal edema*—refers to arytenoid and interarytenoid edema (Fig 4–5).
5. *Posterior commissure hypertrophy*—Swelling of the posterior commissure epithelium, which, with worsening acid injury, can progressively encroach on the airway (Fig 4–6).

Rarely are the signs of LPR seen in isolation, meaning it would be very unusual for a patient to have only a pseudosulcus vocalis as the sole manifestation of LPR. Typically, the patient with LPR has multiple signs of LPR (Fig 4–7) with edema of the larynx, not erythema, being the clinical hallmark of LPR.[7,8]

Laryngopharyngeal Sensory Testing, LPR, and Dysphagia

Traditionally, the diagnosis of LPR is made by a combination of patient history, physical examination of the larynx, and diagnostic in-

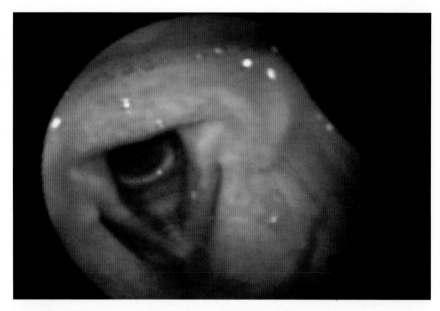

FIGURE 4-3. Normal laryngeal ventricular spacing. Endoscopic view of the hypopharynx in a healthy control demonstrating a 2- to 3-mm opening in the ventricle, the space between the true and false vocal folds.

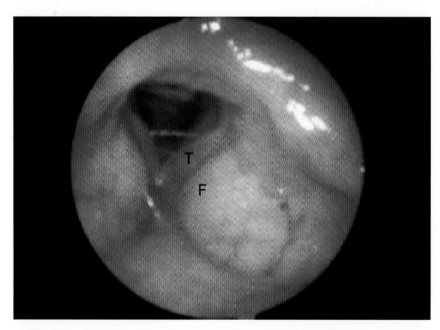

FIGURE 4-4. Ventricle obliteration and true vocal fold edema. The space between the true vocal fold (the letter *T*) and the false vocal folds (the letter *F*) is obliterated—normally there should be approximately 2 to 3 mm of ventricular space between the true vocal folds and the false vocal folds. Also note the polypoid degeneration of the true vocal folds bilaterally.

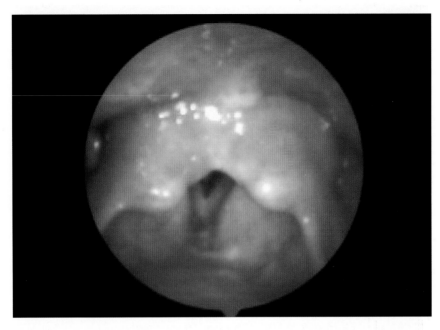

FIGURE 4-5. Diffuse laryngeal edema. There is significant arytenoid and interarytenoid edema so that the posterior half of the airway is obstructed.

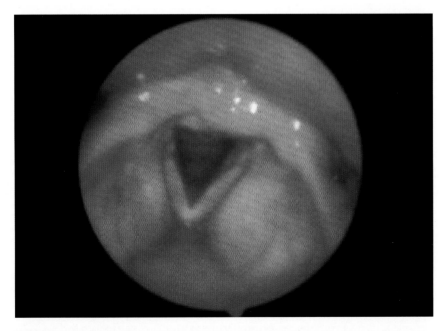

FIGURE 4-6. Posterior commissure hypertrophy. There is edema of the posterior commissure epithelium, which is encroaching on the airway posteriorly.

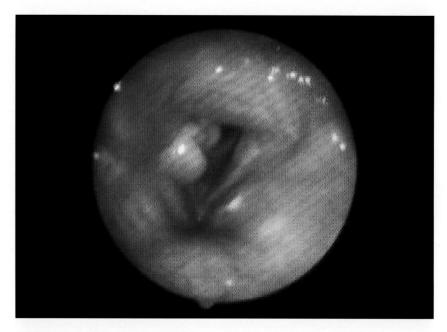

FIGURE 4–7. Stigmata of LPR. Note the presence of multiple signs of LPR. There is a large granuloma along the right vocal process. There are pseudosulcus vocalis, ventricle obliteration, posterior commissure hypertrophy, and marked arytenoid and interarytenoid edema.

strumental testing. Double probe 24-hour pH monitoring is considered to be the most sensitive and specific method of making a diagnosis of LPR.[9] However, patients may not want to have a foreign body in their nose and laryngopharynx for 24 hours in order to be treated for their complaints. Furthermore, the 24-hour pH test is often confounded by the requirement that the patient perform "typical daily activities" while a catheter protrudes out of his or her nose, taped to the cheek. So the patient who starts each day with a cup of coffee, half of a pack of cigarettes, and then some bacon and fried eggs, now gets up, looks in the mirror, sees the catheter coming out of his or her nose, reaches for a glass of water, and then has a teaspoon of yogurt. An in-office, TFL-based test that takes minutes to perform may be much more appealing to a patient.[10]

Among the clinical applications of laryngopharyngeal sensory testing is quantification of the edematous larynx as a result of acid reflux disease. A simple way to look at this is to picture a situation where a clinician sees an edematous arytenoid region (see Fig 4–5) and then imagine that the air pulse strength required to "indent" that area or other areas such as the aryepiglottic fold will be much greater than the air pulse strength necessary to indent normal, non-edematous tissue.

The idea of using laryngopharyngeal sensory testing to quantify the edema that results from LPR has been described in two studies. In one prospective study, LPR was diagnosed by actually witnessing reflux of gastric contents into the hypopharynx during a FEESST.[5] The witnessed reflux events were a result of studying two groups of individuals, patients with dysphagia and healthy age-matched controls. The subjects in both the dysphagia group and the control group drank 30 cc of apple juice containing green food coloring 15 minutes prior to the commencement of the FEESST. If green material was seen presenting itself in the hypopharynx prior to the food administration trials of the FEESST, patients were said to have LPR. The actual study was as follows: FEESST was performed in 54 patients with dysphagia and in 25 healthy controls. The dysphagia group consisted of nonsmokers who had no history of neurologic disease and no rhinitis or sinusitis by history and by CT-scan findings. The dysphagia group was further divided into one of two treatment arms depending on whether or not they were seen to reflux the green apple juice during their initial FEESST. If they were refluxing, this subgroup was called the positive LPR group and were given proton pump inhibitor (PPI) (eg, Omeprazole) therapy for 3 consecutive months, then had a repeat FEESST. The subgroup of dysphagia patients who were not refluxing—no green material seen in the hypopharynx—was called the negative LPR group. They were given a histamine-two (H2) receptor antagonist (eg, ranitidine) for 3 consecutive months and then had a repeat FEESST. The reason the negative LPR group was given an H2-receptor antagonist is that they all had symptoms of LPR, but actual reflux of gastric contents was not observed.

The results indicated that 4% of the control group (one patient) had arytenoid and interarytenoid edema, sensory deficits, and LPR; there were no individuals with erythema. However, the dysphagia group displayed significant differences when compared to the control group. In the dysphagia group, 96% of the patients had arytenoid and interarytenoid edema, 81% had laryngopharyngeal sensory deficits, 70% had LPR, and only 30% had erythema.

The results of the initial FEESST in the dysphagia group showed that half of the patients had severe laryngopharyngeal sensory deficits (LAR elicited at >6.0 mm Hg air pulse pressure) and about half had moderate deficits (4.0–6.0 mm Hg air pulse pressure) or no sensory deficits (LAR elicited at <4.0 mm Hg air pulse pressure). Of the patients with severe deficits, almost all demonstrated laryngeal penetration and one-half of that group aspirated on liquids. In contrast, the moderate-to-no-deficit group rarely demonstrated penetration or aspiration. The differences in incidence of penetration and aspiration between patients with the severe sensory deficits and patients with moderate-to–no-deficit were statistically significant.

After 3 months of treatment with PPI therapy, just prior to the follow-up FEESST, three-quarters of the patients reported that their dysphagia complaints, specifically cough and throat clearing, had resolved. Correspondingly, during the FEESST, edema was noted to have resolved or to be significantly reduced in almost 70% of patients. Furthermore, the laryngeal sensory deficits were improved in about 80% of patients. Most importantly, the incidence of laryngeal penetration and aspiration was significantly less when compared to the pre-PPI treatment FEESST.

Patients in the dysphagia group who were not refluxing, and, therefore, were given H2-receptor antagonists, fared significantly poorer, with dysphagia, cough, and throat clearing persisting in over 75% of cases. During the follow-up FEESST in the H2-receptor antagonist group, patient signs fared no better, with arytenoid and interarytenoid edema persisting in all cases and sensory deficits persisting in 90%.

This study showed that edema is the clinical hallmark of LPR and that this edema can be quantified with laryngopharyngeal sensory testing. Furthermore, patients with dysphagia who reflux during a FEESST have measurable sensory deficits in the posterior larynx. Also, the effect of PPI therapy on the posterior laryngeal edema can be quantified quite precisely.

Another conclusion brought forth by the study is that the posterior laryngeal edema and bilateral severe sensory deficits associated with LPR contribute to significant swallowing abnormalities. These patients have a risk of laryngeal penetration and aspiration at least four times greater than those with no sensory deficits. In addition, treatment of very symptomatic patients with a PPI, versus an H2-receptor antagonist, significantly reduced posterior laryngeal swelling, sensory deficits, and number of untoward swallowing events.

A second prospective controlled study was carried out to examine the relationship between double-probe pH testing, laryngopharyngeal sensory testing, and TFL findings.[11] Seventy-six patients were enrolled in a tightly controlled study. All patients underwent dual channel 24-hour pH testing done 7 days off PPI treatment, laryngopharyngeal sensory testing, and TFL by otolaryngologists who were blinded to pH status and laryngopharyngeal sensory testing results. There were three patient groups: group A (the study group)—patients with GERD who had LPR symptoms; group B (GERD controls)—patients with GERD but no LPR symptoms; group C (normals)—no GERD, no LPR symptoms. GERD was defined as a distal probe pH of less than 4 more than 5.4% of the time over a 24-hour time period.[9]

Patients with GERD and LPR symptoms (group A) had significantly higher posterior laryngopharyngeal sensory thresholds than both patients with GERD but no LPR symptoms and controls with no GERD and no LPR symptoms. Sensitivity of blinded TFL findings versus dual channel 24-hour pH testing was 50%, and specificity was 83%. However, adding laryngopharyngeal sensory thresholds greater than 5 mm Hg air pulse pressure to the TFL findings increased the sensitivity of TFL versus dual probe pH testing from 50% to 88%, and specificity from 83% to 88%.[11]

This study showed that LPR is associated with a posterior laryngeal sensory neuropathy with impairment of the LAR. The investigators reasoned that, because a greater air pulse strength was required to elicit the LAR in the documented acid reflux patients compared to the controls without acid reflux, this finding effectively represented an alteration in laryngeal sensory nerve function, hence their use of the term "neuropathy." Furthermore, adding sensory testing, specifically a sensory deficit greater than 5 mm Hg air pulse pressure, to the TFL findings, was essentially as sensitive and specific as 24-hour pH testing to diagnose acid reflux disease. Practically, what this means for the patient and for the clinician is that a brief in-office test, laryngopharyngeal sensory testing, can serve the same purpose as a 24-hour pH test to diagnose reflux disease. Therefore, these results suggest that with the application of sensory testing techniques identification of reflux disease can be made quite readily by most practicing physicians who see patients with laryngopharyngeal reflux symptoms.

3. SUMMARY

Laryngopharyngeal sensory testing alone provides the clinician with a comprehensive assessment of both the motor and sensory components of laryngeal function. Sensory testing also provides information to separate central neurological deficits from peripheral nerve injuries. In addition, a precise diagnosis of acid reflux disease is possible by correctly interpreting the sensory test findings.

Finally, the use of sensory testing for reflux disease offers an "in the office" immediate diagnosis so that treatment may be initiated at the time of testing.

REFERENCES

1. Reulbach TR, Belafsky PC, Blalock PD, Koufman JA, Postma GN. Occult laryngeal pathology in a community-based cohort. *Otolaryngol Head Neck Surg.* 2001;124:448–450.
2. Koufman J. The otolaryngologic manifestations of gastroesophageal reflux disease (GERD): a clinical investigation of 225 patients using ambulatory 24-hour pH monitoring and an experimental investigation of the role of acid and pepsin in the development of laryngeal injury. *Laryngoscope.* 1991;101(suppl 53):1–78.
3. Shaw GY, Searl JP, Young JL, Miner PB. Subjective, laryngoscopic and acoustic measurements of laryngeal reflux before and after treatment with omeprazole. *J Voice.* 1996;10:410–418.
4. Belafsky PC, Postma GN, Koufman JA. Validity and reliability of the reflux symptom index (RSI). *J Voice.* 2002;16:274–277.
5. Aviv JE, Liu H, Parides M, Kaplan ST, Close LG. Laryngopharyngeal sensory deficits in patients with laryngopharyngeal reflux and dysphagia. *Ann Otol Rhinol Laryngol.* 2000;109:1000–1006.
6. Belafsky PC, Postma GN, Koufman JA. The validity and reliability of the reflux finding score (RFS). *Laryngoscope.* 2001;111:1313–1317.
7. Vaezi MF, Hick DM, Abelson TI, Richter JE. Laryngeal signs and symptoms and gastroesophageal reflux disease (GERD): a critical assessment of cause and effect association. *Clinic Gastroenterol Hepatol.* 2003;1:333–344.
8. Belafsky PC, Postma GN, Amin MR, Koufman JA. Symptoms and findings of laryngopharyngeal reflux. *Ear Nose Throat J.* 2002;81(9 suppl 2):10–13.
9. Richter JE. Diagnostic tests for gastroesophageal reflux disease. *Am J Med Sci.* 2003;326:300–308.
10. Aviv JE, Parides M, Fellowes J, Close LG. Endoscopic evaluation of swallowing as an alternative to 24-hour pH monitoring to diagnose extra-esophageal reflux. *Ann Otol Rhinol Laryngol.* 2000;109(suppl 184):25–27.
11. Botoman VA, Hanft KL, Breno SM, Vickers D, Astor FC, Caristo IB, Alemar GO, Sheth S, Bonner GF. Prospective controlled evaluation of pH testing, laryngoscopy and laryngopharyngeal sensory testing (LPST) shows a specific post inter-arytenoid neuropathy in proximal GERD (P-GERD). LPST improves laryngoscopy diagnostic yield in P-GERD. *Am J Gastroenterol.* 2002;97(9 suppl):S11–S12.

V

Transnasal Esophagoscopy (TNE)

What to Do When the Sensory Test and/or FEESST Results Cannot Explain the Etiology of the Patient's Dysphagia

1. Development and applications of TNE
2. Indications for TNE
3. Technique of TNE
4. Algorithm for when to use TNE, sensory testing, and FEESST
5. What to look for during TNE
6. Summary

INTRODUCTION

What is the next step in the workup of a patient with dysphagia if the laryngopharyngeal portion of the dysphagia investigation is unremarkable? In other words, what should the clinician do if the etiology of the patient's dysphagia complaint is not explainable by the results of the sensory test and the FEESST? The cause of the patient's dysphagia may be pathology in the esophagus or stomach. For instance, esophageal stricture or neoplasm can cause dysphagia. Subtle, but potentially lethal, changes in the esophageal mucosa, which are readily detected during transnasal esophagoscopy (TNE), can be very difficult to see with an esophagram (Fig 5–1).

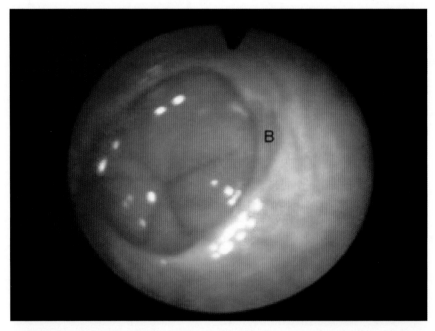

FIGURE 5–1. Short segment Barrett esophagus. Short segment refers to the endoscopic appearance of pink, columnar epithelium in the distal esophagus measuring less than 3 cm in length. In this endoscopic view of the distal esophagus, at 2 o'clock, letter marked "B," there is a sickle-shaped portion of epithelium that is distinctly pink in color and protruding into the gray/white epithelium of the esophagus. This patient did not have heartburn or regurgitation, but was complaining of persistent cough, throat clearing, and excess phlegm, 3 months after taking twice daily PPIs. The biopsy result of this short segment Barrett esophagus was intestinal metaplasia, not the more severe form, dysplasia.

The esophagus can be investigated radiographically with an esophagram or an upper gastrointestinal (GI) series. An endoscopic assessment of the GI tract may also be done. This is known as an upper GI endoscopy, also known as esophagogastroduodenoscopy (EGD).

The esophagus may also be evaluated by transnasal esophagoscopy (TNE). Historically, the technique of transoral rigid esophagoscopy has been a part of the surgical repertoire of the otolaryngologist-head and neck surgeon since the 1890s.[1-3] For the past 40 years rigid esophagoscopy has been performed in the operating room under general anesthesia. On the other hand, flexible esophagoscopy, performed transorally in the endoscopy suite under conscious sedation, has been the domain of the gastroenterologist since the late 1950s. At that time, Basil Hirschowitz, a gastroenterologist, published the first papers on transoral flexible fiberoptic endoscopy of the upper aerodigestive tract.[4,5] Many years later in 1994, Reza Shaker published the first paper on unsedated, transnasal EGD, performed with the patient sitting upright in an examining chair.[6] In 1998, at the annual meeting of the American Broncho-Esophagological Association, an otolaryngologist performed TNE live on a healthy control to demonstrate the ease and reliability of the technique.[7] Since then, TNE has been growing in popularity among otolaryngologists as a vastly safer alternative to traditional conscious sedation flexible esophagoscopy and general anesthesia rigid esophagoscopy.[8-10] In this chapter, the development of TNE is reviewed. The TNE technique is described and indications for its use are presented. Although TNE is not an integral part of FEESST, the need for TNE may derive from the results of the FEESST.

1. DEVELOPMENT AND APPLICATIONS OF TNE

From 1996 to the present, numerous publications in the GI literature have compared unsedated transnasal and sedated transoral upper endoscopy. These studies showed no difference between the two techniques with respect to patient safety, feasibility, and patient tolerance.[11-14] Furthermore, TNE is as accurate as conventional upper endoscopy to detect Barrett esophagus.[15] Most interestingly, very recent work has shown that for patients who have reflux symptoms—heartburn, regurgitation, dysphagia—but do not have other gastric or duodenal symptoms—abdominal pain, nausea, or history of gastric or duodenal ulcer—an endoscopic exam of the esophagus alone (no need to endoscopically examine stomach or duodenum) is sufficient to diagnose the etiology of their complaint.[16]

The reason to examine the esophagus in patients with reflux disease is the demonstrated link between reflux esophagitis and esophageal adenocarcinoma. Reflux esophagitis was first described in 1935.[17] Subsequently, in 1950, Barrett described columnar-lined esophageal epithelium in patients with reflux esophagitis.[18] A few years later, gastroesophageal reflux disease (GERD) was linked to Barrett esophagus.[19] The concept is that GERD can injure the stratified squamous epithelium that normally lines the distal esophagus. When columnar cells, the cell types that line the stomach, replace the reflux-damaged squamous cells, the resulting condition is called Barrett esophagus.[20,21] Endoscopically, Barrett epithelium has a pink appearance, which contrasts rather sharply with the gray/white epithelium of the esophagus (Fig 5–1). In 1975, GERD was linked to Barrett esophagus and esophageal adenocarcinoma.[22]

Since the 1960s esophageal adenocarcinoma has been the most rapidly increasing solid organ tumor in the western world. Specifically, incidence rates for adenocarcinoma in the lower third of the esophagus are unmatched by any other tumor.[23,24] The incidence of adenocarcinoma of the esophagus has increased by 350% over the past 30 years in white men and 300% in white women.[24-26] The risk factors for esophageal adenocarcinoma are presence of Barrett esophagus and gastroesophageal (GE) reflux. The potential public health problem is enormous as GERD affects 40% of adults in the United States.[27] Furthermore, Barrett esophagus develops in 5 to 20% of patients with GERD and, as mentioned, predisposes to esophageal adenocarcinoma.[28]

Most cases of esophageal adenocarcinoma are detected when the cancer is advanced and incurable with the 5-year survival rates of symptomatic esophageal adenocarcinoma less than 10%.[29,30] Systematic endoscopic biopsy can detect adenocarcinoma of the esophagus at an early stage with the 5-year survival rate increasing to 80 to 90% as a result of early detection.[31] Therefore, endoscopic surveillance is recommended for early detection of adenocarcinoma in patients with Barrett esophagus.[31]

A solution to the dismal survival after diagnosis of symptomatic esophageal adenocarcinoma may be more frequent upper GI endoscopies. One of the reasons this is not done routinely is that conscious, or intravenous, sedation, typically has been required for upper endoscopy. Most complications related to EGD result from conscious sedation, with cardiopulmonary events comprising more than 60% of all major complications.[32] Conscious sedation may result in oversedation, hypoxemia, arrhythmia, and vasovagal reaction. Intravenous sedation has been shown to be the most common independent risk factor for the development of negative outcomes within 30 days of outpatient upper GI endoscopy.[33,34]

Unsedated TNE necessarily obviates the primary source of complications—intravenous sedation—related to upper GI endoscopy and consequently removes a major stumbling block to frequent, routine endoscopic surveillance of the esophagus. Imagine a clinical environment where endoscopic examination of the esophagus can take place as readily and as free of complications as a transnasal flexible laryngoscopy. Patients' esophageal lesions will likely be detected when early, small, and asymptomatic rather than when late, large, and symptomatic. It is highly likely that TNE will profoundly improve the incidence of early diagnosis of asymptomatic adenocarcinoma of the esophagus and ultimately lead to improved survival of this disease.

2. INDICATIONS FOR TNE

Should everyone with heartburn undergo a TNE? Probably not. However, patients with persistent laryngopharyngeal reflux (LPR) symptoms represent a different, higher risk group of patients than typical GERD patients with heartburn. Recent work has shown that persistent LPR symptoms, especially cough, may herald esophageal adenocarcinoma with greater reliability than typical GERD symptoms.[35] Therefore, we generally recommend TNE for patients with persistent LPR symptoms despite antacid therapy, and for patients with dysphagia complaints when the laryngopharyngeal exam—FEESST and sensory testing alone—cannot explain the etiology of the patients' dysphagia complaints.

3. TECHNIQUE OF TNE

The keys to successful completion of a TNE are adequate topical nasal anesthesia and nasal decongestion. In addition, the patient should not eat nor drink for at least 3 hours before the TNE, so that the stomach is empty before the exam. No conscious or intravenous sedation is used. We generally spray 1% lidocaine with epinephrine 1:100,000 in the nose and 20% benzocaine in the oropharynx. It is very important to use only a small amount of oropharyngeal anesthesia because the patient's ability to swallow on demand is critical to successful performance of a TNE. If the patient's laryngopharynx is too numb from an excess of topical oropharyngeal anesthesia, he or she will be intermittently aspirating secretions and not have enough sensory feedback from the hypopharynx to swallow air or saliva when asked.

Two different types of TNE systems are available. One system is a video-chip flexible endoscope where the camera is located on the distal tip of the endoscope and the proximal portion of the scope is attached to a video processor (Pentax; Olympus) (Fig 5–2). The video-chip endoscope has a working channel built within the scope, which allows passage of air, water, suction, and 1.8 mm biopsy instruments. The other system is an add-on camera flexible endoscope in which a camera is attached to the proximal portion of the fiberscope, usually at the eyepiece (Fig 5–3). The fiberoptic add-on camera system can incorporate a single-use disposable TNE endosheath (Medtronic-Xomed; Vision Sciences) (Fig 5–4). The TNE endosheath has one channel for air insufflation and/or suction and is used primarily as a diagnostic, as opposed to a therapeutic, in-

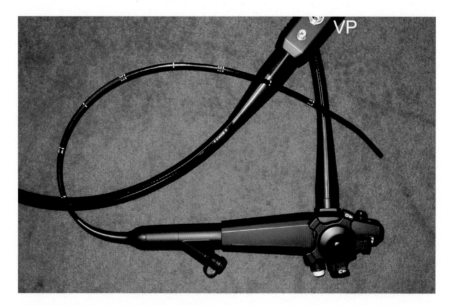

FIGURE 5–2. Video-chip TNE endoscope. This is a single wheel distal video-chip endoscope. The portion of the endoscope that is placed in the video processor is marked VP.

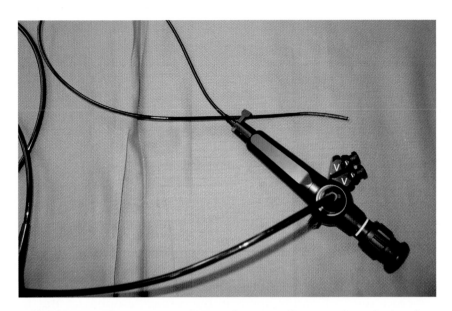

FIGURE 5–3. Add-on camera TNE endoscope. There are two pinch valves (v) protruding from the scope, one is for air insufflation and the other is for suction.

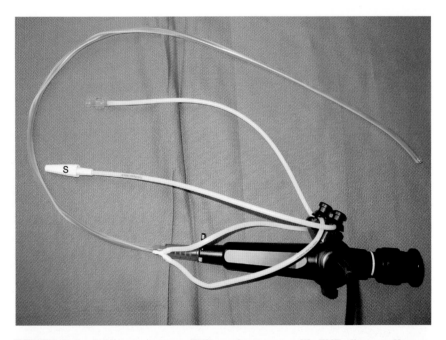

FIGURE 5–4. Add-on camera TNE endoscope with TNE diagnostic endosheath. The diagnostic TNE endosheath has been placed on the add-on camera TNE endoscope. The catheter allowing suction to take place is marked "S." The other catheter is used to insufflate air into the esophagus.

strument. A therapeutic TNE scope and endosheath system (Fig 5–5), which contains a biopsy channel that allows passage of a 1.8 mm cup forceps (Figs 5–6 and 5–7), is also available.

There are two ways of passing the TNE scope through the patient's cricopharyngeus. In one technique, the patient is asked to burp. During the actual burp, the cricopharyngeus opens and the TNE scope can be readily passed posterior to the cricoid into the cervical esophagus (Fig 5–8). In the other technique, the patient is asked to tuck his or her chin to the chest and then to swallow saliva. The TNE endoscope should be hovering over the postcricoid region anticipating the onset of a swallow. As the laryngohyoid complex moves superiorly and anteriorly, the cricopharyngeus snaps open and the esophagus is then readily intubated. The hovering then swallow technique is the one most clinicians use because the burp-on-command technique is too difficult for most patients to perform.

Once the TNE endoscope is in the cervical esophagus, the examiner should follow the peristaltic wave distally ("ride the peristaltic wave") as the esophageal lumen slowly opens and the swallowed air bolus propagates distally toward the esophagogastric (EG) junction.

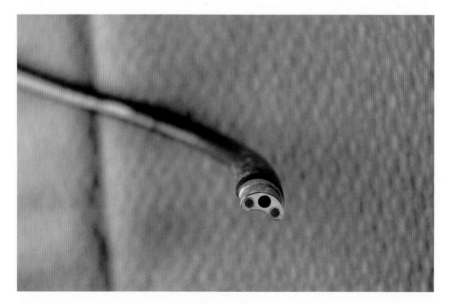

FIGURE 5–5. D-shaped TNE endoscope. Unusual design of a flexible endoscope that allows for an ultrathin diameter.

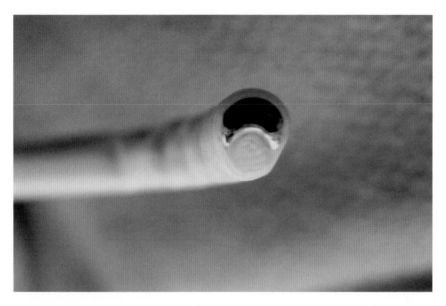

FIGURE 5-6. D-shaped TNE endoscope scope with endosheath loaded. The endosheath is now loaded on the D-shaped scope showing the 2.1 mm in diameter working channel.

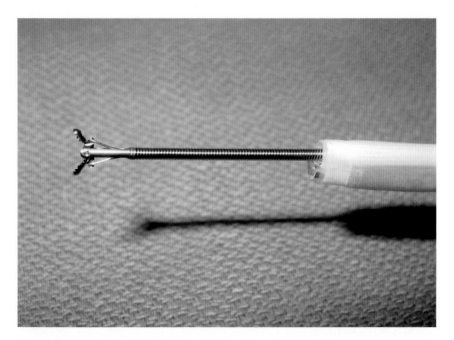

FIGURE 5-7. TNE endosheath with biopsy capability. Cup forceps is protruding through distal portion of the working channel of a single-use disposable TNE endosheath loaded on the D-shaped endoscope.

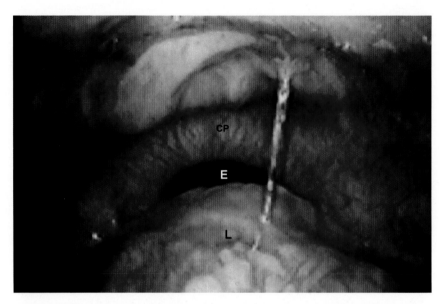

FIGURE 5–8. Cricopharyngeal opening. Endoscopic view of cricopharyngeal (CP) muscle "snapping" open as a patient is burping. This is also the view one would see at the moment of the swallow where the cricopharyngeus opens as the larynx (L) is lifting away from the posterior pharyngeal wall effectively exposing the cervical esophagus (E).

4. ALGORITHM FOR WHEN TO USE TNE, SENSORY TESTING, AND FEESST

TNE is not a replacement for FEESST, nor is it a part of the FEESST examination. It is a separate examination of the esophagus. How does the clinician begin to use information regarding TNE, sensory testing, or FEESST to decide when to use each test? We have developed an algorithm that allows clinicians to decide when to use TNE and when to use sensory testing and FEESST (Fig 5–9). The key in determining what test to perform initially depends on the nature of the patient's complaint. If the patient is complaining of a swallowing problem, or dysphagia, one should start with a FEESST. If the FEESST is unremarkable, that is, the laryngopharyngeal exam is normal and no sensory deficits are detected, then the source of the dysphagia is likely in the esophagus and a TNE is indicated.

If the patient is not complaining of dysphagia, but rather is complaining of LPR symptoms—cough, hoarseness, throat clearing, excess phlegm—then we recommend that the patient workup start with a laryngopharyngeal sensory test, which always includes

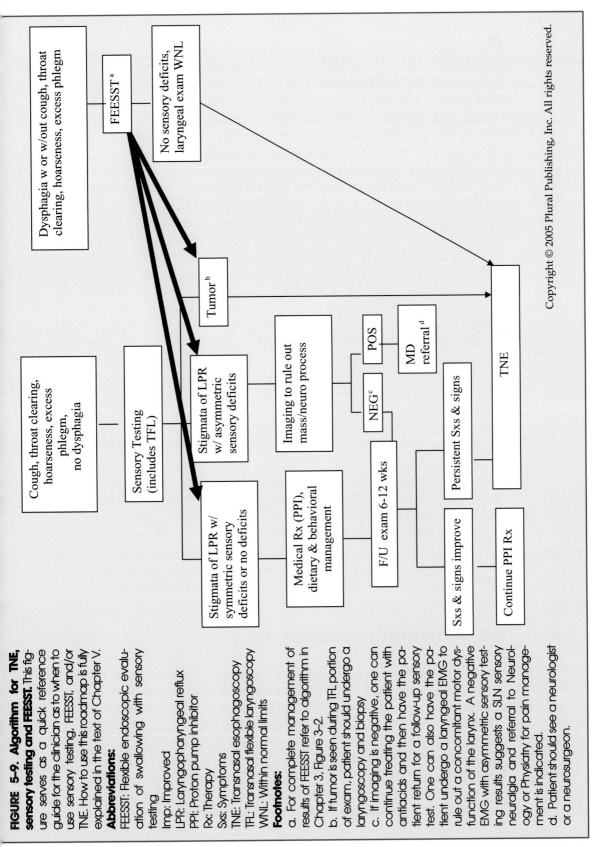

FIGURE 5-9. Algorithm for TNE, sensory testing and FEESST. This figure serves as a quick reference guide for the clinician as to when to use sensory testing, FEESST, and/or TNE. How to use this roadmap is fully explained in the text of Chapter V.

Abbreviations:

FEESST: Flexible endoscopic evaluation of swallowing with sensory testing
Imp: Improved
LPR: Laryngopharyngeal reflux
PPI: Proton pump inhibitor
Rx: Therapy
Sxs: Symptoms
TNE: Transnasal esophagoscopy
TFL: Transnasal flexible laryngoscopy
WNL: Within normal limits

Footnotes:

a. For complete management of results of FEESST refer to algorithm in Chapter 3, Figure 3-2.

b. If tumor is seen during TFL portion of exam, patient should undergo a laryngoscopy and biopsy.

c. If imaging is negative, one can continue treating the patient with antiacids and then have the patient return for a follow-up sensory test. One can also have the patient undergo a laryngeal EMG to rule out a concomitant motor dysfunction of the larynx. A negative EMG with asymmetric sensory testing results suggests a SLN sensory neuralgia and referral to Neurology or Physiatry for pain management is indicated.

d. Patient should see a neurologist or a neurosurgeon.

Dysphagia w or w/out cough, throat clearing, hoarseness, excess phlegm

FEESST [a]

No sensory deficits, laryngeal exam WNL

Tumor [b]

Cough, throat clearing, hoarseness, excess phlegm, no dysphagia

Sensory Testing (includes TFL)

Stigmata of LPR w/ asymmetric sensory deficits

Stigmata of LPR w/ symmetric sensory deficits or no deficits

Imaging to rule out mass/neuro process

NEG [c]

POS

MD referral [d]

Medical Rx (PPI), dietary & behavioral management

F/U exam 6-12 wks

Persistent Sxs & signs

Sxs & signs improve

TNE

Continue PPI Rx

a transnasal flexible laryngoscopy (TFL). If the sensory test shows stigmata of LPR (pseudosulcus vocalis, ventricle obliteration, arytenoid and interarytenoid edema)—no matter what the sensory test shows (as long as the test result is symmetric)—the patient likely has LPR and should be treated with reflux precautions and antacid therapy, typically proton pump inhibitors (PPIs). However, if LPR signs are present and the patient has asymmetric sensory deficits, meaning the sensory thresholds are different from the right to the left side of the laryngopharynx, a different type of workup must ensue. Imaging of the brain and neck should be done to rule out a mass in the brain or along the course of the vagus nerve, as well as to rule out a cerebrovascular process intracranially. If the imaging is positive, the patient is referred to neurology or neurosurgery. If the imaging is negative, there are several avenues to take. One approach is to continue treating the patient with a vigorous antacid regimen and have the patient return for a follow-up sensory test. Another approach is to send the patient for a laryngeal EMG to rule out a concomitant motor dysfunction of the larynx. A negative EMG with asymmetric sensory testing results suggests an SLN sensory neuralgia and referral to neurology or physiatry for management of neuralgia would be indicated.

If, at any time during a FEESST or a sensory test, a mass is seen in the laryngopharynx, plans must be made for a biopsy of the lesion. Often, an esophagoscopy is indicated as well, to rule out a synchronous lesion in the esophagus. With the advent of TNE endoscopes and channeled TFL scopes (or standard TFL scopes with biopsy endosheaths), laryngoscopy with biopsy and esophagoscopy with biopsy can now be performed in the office under topical anesthesia, thereby avoiding the patient's risk and time consumption inherent in operating room procedures performed under general anesthesia.

5. WHAT TO LOOK FOR DURING TNE

Several portions of the TNE require particular attention. One is the postcricoid region and the proximal cervical esophagus. This region is very difficult to visualize during a standard EGD. One can overcome this difficulty during a TNE by video-recording the TNE procedure. This allows the physician to review the images and to "freeze frame" the instant where the cricopharyngeus muscle snaps open as the swallow is initiated. By capturing that moment, one can see the entire cricopharyngeal region in its circumference and thereby rule out a mass in this area (see Fig 5–8). The other region that requires especially careful review and scrutiny is the GE junction, in particular the area of the Z-line, where the gray/white squamous epithelium of the esophagus ends and the pink, salmon-colored columnar epithelium of the stomach begins (Fig 5–10). Again, we recommend a freeze frame of the GE junction so that Barrett esophagus or other pathology can be detected.

6. SUMMARY

TNE is performed in the physician's office without the sophisticated patient monitoring and skilled ancillary personnel that are required for flexible esophagoscopy using conscious sedation in the endoscopy suite or rigid esophagoscopy using general anesthesia in the operating room. Moving to the office setting reduces overall health care costs and directly enhances the efficiency and productivity of the clinician. As otolaryngologists get reacquainted with the esophagus, their most important responsibility will be to match their expertise in the diagnosis and management of hypopharyngeal disease with that of esophageal disease.

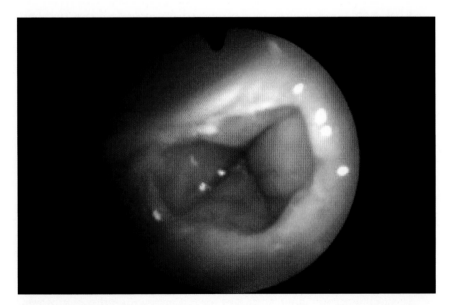

FIGURE 5-10. Z-line. The Z-line represents the area of the distal esophagus where the gray/white squamous epithelium of the esophagus ends and the pink, salmon-colored columnar epithelium of the stomach begins.

REFERENCES

1. Jackson C. *The Life of Chevalier Jackson. An Autobiography.* New York, NY: Macmillan; 1938.
2. Moore I. Peroral endoscopy: an historical survey from its origin to the present day. *J Laryngol Otol.* 1926;41:277–298.
3. Marsh BR. Historic development of bronchoesophagology. *Otolaryngol Head Neck Surg.* 1996;114:689–716.
4. Hirschowitz BI, Curtiss LE, Peters CW, Pollard HM. Demonstration of a new gastroscope "the fiberscope." *Gastroenterology.* 1958;35:50–53.
5. Hirschowitz BI. A fibre optic flexible oesophagoscope. *Lancet.* 1963; 2:388.
6. Shaker, R. Unsedated trans-nasal pharyngoesophagogastroduodenoscopy (t-EGD). *Gastrointest Endosc.* 1994;40:346–348.
7. Aviv JE, Takoudes T, Ma G, Close LG. Office-based esophagoscopy—a preliminary report. *Otolaryngol Head Neck Surg.* 2001;125:170–175.
8. Postma GN, Bach KK, Belafsky PC, Koufman JA. The role of transnasal esophagoscopy in head and neck oncology. *Laryngoscope.* 2002; 112:2242–2243.
9. Koufman JA, Belafsky PC, Bach KK, Daniel E, Postma GN. Prevalence of esophagitis in patients with pH-documented laryngopharyngeal reflux. *Laryngsocope.* 2002;112:1606–1609.
10. Belafsky PC. Office endoscopy for the laryngologist/bronchoesophagologist. *Curr Opin Otolaryngol Head Neck Surg.* 2002;10:467–471.
11. Catanzaro A, Faulx AL, Isenberg GA, Wong K, Cooper G, Sivak MV, Chak A. Prospective evaluation of 4 mm diameter endoscopes for esophagoscopy in sedated and unsedated patients. *Gastrointest Endosc.* 2003; 57;300–304.
12. Faulx AL, Catanzaro A, Zyzanski S, Cooper GS, Pfau PR, Isenberg G, Wong RCK, Sivak MV, Chak A. Patient tolerance and acceptance of unsedated ultrathin endoscopy. *Gastrointest Endosc.* 2002;55:620–623.
13. Zaman A, Hahn M, Hapke R, Knigge K, Fennerty BM, Katon RM. A randomized trial of peroral versus transnasal endscopy using ultrathin video endoscope. *Gastrointest Endosc.* 1999;49:279–284.
14. Mokhashi MS, Wildi SM, Glenn TF, Wallace MB, Jost C, Gumustop B, Kim CY, Cotton PB, Hawes RH. A prospective, blinded study of diagnostic esophagoscopy with a superthin, stand-alone, battery-powered esophagoscope. *Am J Gastroenterol.* 2003;98:2383–2389.
15. Saeian K, Staff DM, Vasilopoulos S, Townsend WF, Almagro UA, Komorowski RA, Choi H, Shaker R. Unsedated transnasal endoscopy accurately detects Barrett's metaplasia and dysplasia *Gastrointest Endosc.* 2002;56:472–478.
16. Wildi SM, Glenn TF, Woolson RF, Wang W, Hawes RH, Wallace MB. Is esophagoscopy alone sufficient for patients with reflux symptoms? *Gastrointest Endosc.* 2004;59:349–354.
17. Winkelstein A. Peptic esophagitis: a new clinical entity. *JAMA.* 1935; 104:906–909.

18. Barrett NR. Chronic peptic ulcer of the oesophagus and "oesophagitis." *Br J Surg.* 1950;38:175–182.

19. Allison PR, Johnstone AS. The oesophagus lined with gastric mucosa membrane. *Thorax.* 1953;8:87–101.

20. Morales CP, Spechler SJ. Intestinal metaplasia at the gastroesophageal junction: Barrett's, bacteria and biomarkers. *Am J Gastroenterol.* 2003; 98:759–762.

21. Spechler SJ, Goyal RK. The columnar lined esophagus, intestinal metaplasia, and Norman Barrett. *Gastroenterology.* 1996;110:614–621.

22. Naef AP, Savary M, Ozzello L. Columnar-lined lower esophagus: an acquired lesion with malignant predisposition. Report on 140 cases of Barrett's esophagus with 12 adenocarcnimoas. *J Thorac Cardiovasc Surg.* 1975;70:826–835.

23. Kocher HM, Patel S, Linklater K, Ellul JP. Increase in incidence of oesophagosgastric carcinoma in the south Thames region: an epidemiological study. *Br J Surg.* 2000;87:362–373.

24. Brock MV, Gou M, Akiyama Y, Muller A, Wu TT, Montgomery E, Deasel M, Germonpre P, Rubinson L, Heitmiller RF, Yang SC, Forastiere AA, Baylin SB, Herman JG. Prognostic importance of promoter hypermethylation of multiple genes in esophageal adenocarcinoma. *Clin Cancer Res.* 2003;9:2912–2919.

25. Devea SS, Blot WJ, Fraumeni JF. Changing patterns in the incidence of esophageal and gastric carcinoma in the United States. *Cancer.* 1998;83:2049–2053.

26. Reid BJ, Blount PL, Rabinovitch PS. Biomarkers in Barrett's esophagus. *Gastrointest Endosc Clin North Am.* 2003; 13:369–397.

27. Locke GR III, Talley NJ, Fett SL, Zinsmeister AR, Melton LJ III. Prevalence and clinical spectrum of gastroesophageal reflux: a population-based study in Olmstead county, Minnesota. *Gastroenterology.* 1997;112:1448–1456.

28. Spechler SJ, Zeroogian JM, Antonioli DA, Wang HH, Goyal RK. Prevalence of metaplasia at the gastro-oesophageal junction. *Lancet.* 1994;344:1533–1536.

29. Lund O, Kimose HH, Aagard MT, Hasenkam JM, Erlandsen M. Risk stratification and long-term results after surgical treatment of carcinoma of the thoracic esophagus and cardia. A 25-year retrospective study. *J Thorac Cardiovasc Surg.* 1990;99:200–209.

30. Farrow DC, Vaughn TL. Determinants of survival following the diagnosis of esophageal adenocarcinoma (United States). *Cancer Causes Control.* 1996;7:322–327.

31. Peters JH, Clark GW, Ireland AP, Chandrasoma P, Smyrk TC, DeMeester TR. Outcome of adenocarcinoma arising in Barrett's esophagus in endoscopically surveyed and nonsurveyed patients. *J Thorac Cardiovasc Surg.* 1994;108:813–821.

32. Chan MF. Complications of upper gastrointestinal endoscopy. *Gastrointest Endosc Clin North Am.* 1996;6:287–303.

33. Fleischer DE, Van de Mierop F, Eisen GM, Al Kawas FH, Benjamin SB, Lewis JH, Nguyen CC, Avigan M, Tio TL, Kidwell JA. A new system for defining endoscopic complications emphasizing the measure of importance. *Gastrointest Endosc.* 1997;45:128–133.
34. Bini EJ, Firoozi B, Rosa J, Choung, RJ, Eyad M, Ali, EM, Osman M, Weinshel EH. Systematic evaluation of complications related to endoscopy in a training setting: a prospective 30-day outcomes study. *Gastrointest Endosc.* 2003;57:8–16.
35. Reavis KM, Morris CD, Gopal DV, Hunter JG, Jobe BA. Laryngopharyngeal reflux symptoms better predict the presence of esophageal adenocarcinoma than typical gastroesophageal reflux symptoms. *Ann Surg.* 2004;239:849–856.

VI

FEESST Safety

INTRODUCTION

FEESST is routinely performed with a team involving a physician and a speech-language pathologist (SLP). In the broadest terms, the physician is present during the FEESST examination to make medical diagnoses. The physician's role is to rule in or to rule out anatomic and physiologic abnormalities of the oral and nasal cavities as well as the nasopharynx, oropharynx, and laryngopharynx.

The role of the SLP is to assess lip and tongue strength, tongue range of motion, and the communication skills of the patient. In addition, the SLP determines what modalities of speech and swallowing therapies, if any, can be applied to increase the safety of swallowing and to maintain nutrition. The American Academy of Otolaryngology–Head and Neck Surgery has written a policy statement regarding endoscopy for swallowing, under which FEESST and sensory testing fall. The policy details the general "division of labor" among physicians and SLPs with respect to endoscopy for swallowing (Fig 6–1). The statement is not a law and in some states it has been superseded by state regulations. Rather, it is a framework within which the group of specialists most often involved in swallowing evaluations generally works. Physicians and SLPs should always consult their state review boards to determine the limitations and scope of practice each examiner plays in FEESST assessment.

1. RESEARCH ON FEESST SAFETY

Passing a thin, flexible endoscope into the widest area of the pharynx intuitively seems to be safe, and this has been proven in initial studies of FEESST safety.[1,2] However, there are areas of the United States where an SLP, supervised by a physician, is not permitted to perform endoscopic swallowing tests. These states usually cite concerns about patient safety.[3,4] However, those concerns for patient safety during a FEESST are not supported by the published data.

From a review of the three largest studies of FEESST safety, a picture emerges of an extraordinarily safe procedure.[1,2,5] A safe FEESST procedure is defined as having a low incidence of epistaxis (nosebleed), changes in heart rate, and airway compromise. In addition, patient comfort is germane to any procedure involving an awake patient. The concern for discomfort is that endoscopic procedures that cause discomfort may cause the patient to move excessively during the procedure or remove the endoscope too rapidly

Fiberoptic Endoscopic Examinations of Swallowing

Fiberoptic endoscopy is an imaging procedure that may be utilized by qualified health care providers (upon direct authorization of a physician) to evaluate velopharyngeal, phonatory, and swallowing functions in adults and children. Physicians are the only professionals qualified and licensed to render medical diagnoses related to the identification of pathology affecting swallowing functions.

Consequently, examinations should be viewed and interpreted by an otolaryngologist or other physician with training in this procedure. In addition, otolaryngologists or other physicians with training in this procedure should directly supervise non-physician professionals who are performing this procedure.

Fiberoptic endoscopy may also be utilized as a therapeutic aid and biofeedback tool during the conduct of swallowing therapy. Care should be taken to use this examination only in settings that ensure patient safety.

Approved: March, 2003

Guidelines are not a substitute for the experience and judgment of a physician and are developed to enhance the physicians' ability to practice evidence-based medicine.

Important Notice

The American Academy of Otolaryngology-Head and Neck Surgery, Inc. and Foundation (AAO-HNS/F) Policy Statements are guidelines only. In no sense do they represent a standard of care. The applicability of an indicator for a procedure, and/or of the process or outcome criteria, must be determined by the responsible physician in light of all the circumstances presented by the individual patient. Adherence to these guidelines will not ensure successful treatment in every situation. The AAO-HNS emphasizes that these policies should not be deemed inclusive of all proper treatment decisions or methods of care, nor exclusive of other treatment decisions or methods of care reasonably directed to obtaining the same results.

FIGURE 6-1. Position statement of the American Academy of Otolaryngology—Head and Neck Surgery (AAO-HNS) on endoscopy for swallowing. (Reprinted with the permission if the American Academy of Otolaryngology—Head and Neck Surgery Foundation.)

and cause nasal trauma. In addition, patient discomfort during a swallowing procedure may prevent the examiner from completing the examination.

In 2000, Aviv et al reported on 500 FEESST examinations performed on 253 inpatients and outpatients seen over a 2½-year period.[1] The purpose of the study was to determine the safety and comfort of the FEESST procedure. The study group had a variety of underlying diagnoses, with the largest cohort being poststroke (48%) and the second largest group being those with chronic neurological diseases (33%). The FEESST examinations were performed by physicians or speech-language pathologists who had performed at least 50 FEESST exams previously.

In a somewhat different population, in 2003, Cohen and colleagues assessed FEESST safety on 349 FEESST examinations conducted on 305 patients in an outpatient setting.[2] The underlying diagnoses ranged from stroke to laryngopharyngeal reflux (LPR) disease. In this study, safety parameters, indicated by incidence of epistaxis, heart rate changes, and airway compromise, were monitored and recorded prior to and following the examination. In addition, patients were asked to rate their level of comfort/discomfort during the exam.

Subsequently, in 2004, a larger cohort of patients with swallowing disorders was examined by Aviv and colleagues in an effort to identify safety and comfort factors related to FEESST in inpatient and outpatients.[5] The largest subgroup was again poststroke patients (25.6%); however, surprisingly, the second largest group was cardiac related (22.2%), followed by a group with head and neck cancer-related swallowing disorders (15.4%).

In these three FEESST safety papers published over an 8-year period, 2,189 FEESST evaluations were performed in 1,634 patients, both inpatients and outpatients. The incidence of epistaxis was 9/2,189 (0.4%). There were no instances of airway compromise in 2,189 cases. There was no statistically significant difference between the average pre- and post-test heart rates. Furthermore, no patients became symptomatically bradycardic or tachycardic.

Of the patients having the cognitive ability to respond to questions regarding the relative degree of comfort/discomfort of the FEESST, the following was noted: Of the 1990 patients reporting, no discomfort was seen in 222 patients (11.0%); mild discomfort was noted in 1077 patients (54.1%); moderate discomfort was noted in 528 (26.5%); and severe discomfort was reported in 63 patients (8.2%).

Of the patients able to respond to whether or not they would repeat the FEESST (n = 1990), 1818 patients (95.7%) said they would repeat the FEESST. Finally, the FEESST was completed in 2140 of 2189 patients (97.8%). This is especially noteworthy because, for most patients, multiple consistencies of liquids and foods are administered to identify problems related to patient complaints.

2. FEESST SAFETY AND DYSPHAGIA ETIOLOGIES

When analyzing the underlying diagnoses that led to the FEESST examination, one must distinguish between the outpatient and inpatient populations. The most common diagnosis in the outpatient setting is LPR (46%), followed, in decreasing order, by stroke, chronic neurodegenerative disease, and then head and neck cancer. With inpatients, stroke is the most common reason for the FEESST, for slightly more than 25% of patients. The second most common reason for a FEESST evaluation in the inpatient population, with slightly less than 25% of patients, is a group that previously was not recognized as a common etiology of dysphagia, namely, cardiac-related diagnoses. The majority of cardiac-related cases in the acute, inpatient setting occur following open-heart surgery (almost 60% of cases), followed by heart attack, congestive heart failure, and new arrhythmia.

What is it about open-heart surgery that might predispose patients to dysphagia? To address this question one must look at a previous study that examined the incidence of dysphagia after open-heart surgery. The study demonstrated two factors that increase dysphagia risk after open-heart surgery: age greater than 65 years and use of transesophageal echocardiography (TE).[6] TE involves the passage of a large caliber instrument via the mouth into the esophagus. It is performed during almost every open-heart operation and can be traumatic to the laryngopharynx.[7] Another likely reason for dysphagia in the post-cardiac surgery, non-CVA cohort is untreated acid reflux disease.[8] In the most recent FEESST safety publication, the post-cardiac surgery, non-CVA group of patients had either moderate or severe sensory deficits in almost 90% of cases. Recent work has shown that sensory deficits greater than 5 mm Hg air pulse pressure is nearly 90% sensitive and 90% specific as a diagnostic indicator of reflux disease when compared with 24-hour pH testing.[9] Therefore, it is quite possible that the etiology of dysphagia in the post-cardiac surgery patients was at least partially due to untreated, or insufficiently treated, acid reflux disease.

FEESST is performed in an effort to maximize the safety of the swallow and, in so doing, maximize patients' opportunity of sustaining themselves with oral intake of food. The overall incidence of untoward events during a FEESST is very small when examining the safety studies. Patient discomfort is the most common potential finding; however, even patients with severe discomfort reported that they would be willing to take the exam again. The finding of discomfort during a FEESST is not unexpected because generally no topical anesthesia is administered to the nasal mucosa during the exam. Given that more than 97% of FEESST evaluations are successfully completed, the transient discomfort engendered by having a small flexible endoscope in the nose and oropharynx appeared to have been acceptable to almost all the patients studied. Our results regarding patient tolerance of flexible laryngoscopy without topical anesthesia corroborate the findings of previous work demonstrating no significant differences in patient comfort level when patients were randomized to topical anesthesia, a vasoconstrictor, or a placebo just before a transnasal flexible laryngoscopy.[10]

3. FEESST SAFETY AND POSSIBLE COMPLICATIONS

The potential complication of FEESST that strikes fear in every clinician is laryngospasm. However, this fear is misguided. When FEESST is properly performed, laryngospasm should not occur. Laryngospasm, defined as sustained adduction of the aryepiglottic folds, false and true vocal folds, does not take place in an awake individual as long as the true vocal folds are not vigorously manipulated.[11,12] However, in patients awakening from general anesthesia, laryngospasm can occur if almost any portion of the endolarynx is manipulated.[13,14] As a rule, FEESST is not performed on patients in the immediate postoperative period while recovering from general anesthesia. Our experience with thousands of cases supports our belief that laryngospasm from FEESST is a hypothetical concern rather than a real issue. In the three studies that reported on patient safety, there were no instances of laryngospasm.[1,2,5]

Nosebleeds occurred in less than 0.5% of patients studied. One would actually anticipate a greater incidence of epistaxis because patients with a history of embolic stroke are usually placed on some type of anticoagulant. Nonetheless, in the day-to-day reality of clinical practice, passage of a small-caliber flexible endoscope, under direct vision in a magnified field, is a technical endeavor that can be performed without significant trauma to the nasal mucosa.

Vasovagal responses have not been reported in the FEESST safety literature. Nevertheless, the possibility of a vasovagal reaction exists in any situation in which an individual may be exposed to anxiety, emotional stress, or severe pain.[15] Therefore, in the setting of FEESST evaluations, constant patient reassurance by a calm, relaxed, comfortable clinician—vocal local (calm, reassuring voice)—can be helpful in preventing a vasovagal event.

In the combined published series assessing changes in heart rate in patients undergoing FEESST, no significant changes in heart rate were found after the procedure compared with heart rate before the procedure. In general, one would only expect a significant change in heart rate if the laryngopharyngeal tissues were handled to the extent that they are during endotracheal intubation.[16,17]. A 3.4-mm-diameter flexible laryngoscope simply cannot exert the same type of stretching forces as a rigid laryngoscope blade. Therefore, significant changes in heart rate would be surprising when a thin flexible endoscope is positioned in the widest portion of the laryngopharynx.

The group of patients that appeared to have the most difficulty with FEESST was the group of patients with advanced amyotrophic lateral sclerosis (ALS). One explanation for this finding is the hyperreflexia and exaggerated frontal release signs seen in such patients.[18] This does not preclude ALS patients from having a FEESST, but it simply means that the physician may require more assistance with patient positioning and reassurance than with non-ALS patients.

4. SUMMARY

When FEESST is performed by trained clinicians, it is an extremely safe method to assess swallowing function. The published FEESST safety data support the premise that FEESST can be performed safely when carried out by highly trained SLPs working with a physician. The concerns for patient safety described by a few are not borne out in carefully controlled studies of FEESST swallow safety. When FEESST is performed according to the protocol described in Chapter II by properly trained clinicians, the incidence of complications is practically nonexistent.

REFERENCES

1. Aviv JE, Kaplan ST, Thompson JE, Spitzer J, Diamond B, Close, LG. The safety of flexible endoscopic evaluation of swallowing with sensory testing (FEESST): an analysis of 500 consecutive evaluations. *Dysphagia*. 2000;15:39–44.

2. Cohen MA, Setzen M, Perlman PW, Ditkoff M, Mattucci KF, Guss J. The safety of flexible endoscopic evaluation of swallowing with sensory testing in an outpatient otolaryngology setting. *Laryngoscope.* 2003;113:21–24.

3. McClure, PS. New Jersey Department of Law and Public Safety, Division of Consumer Affairs. Audiology and Speech-Language Pathology Advisory Committee Public Session Minutes of November 8, 2001. Available at: http://www.state.nj.us/lps/ca/aud/minutes/audio118.htm

4. Special Notice Audiology and Speech-Language Pathology Advisory Committee, New Jersey Department of Law and Public Safety, Division of Consumer Affairs. Accessed Feb 2003. Available at: http://www.state.nj.us/lps/ca/aud/fees.htm

5. Aviv JE. Murry T, Zschommler A, Cohen M, Gartner C. Flexible endoscopic evaluation of swallowing with sensory testing: patient characteristics and analysis of safety in 1340 consecutive examinations. *Ann Otol Rhinol Laryngol.* 2005;114:173–176.

6. Rousou JA, Tighe DA, Garb JL, Krasner H, Engelman RM, Flack JE III, Deaton DW. Risk of dysphagia after transesophageal echocardiography during cardiac operations. *Ann Thorac Surg.* 2000;69:486–489.

7. Aviv JE, DiTullio MR, Homma S, Storper IS, Zschommier A, Ma G, Petkova E, Murphy M, Desloge R, Shaw G, Benjamin S, Corwin S. Hypopharyngeal perforation near-miss during transesophageal echocardiography. *Laryngoscope.* 2004;114:821–826.

8. Aviv JE, Liu H, Parides M, Kaplan ST, Close LG. Laryngopharyngeal sensory deficits in patients with laryngopharyngeal reflux and dysphagia. *Ann Otol Rhinol Laryngol.* 2000;109:1000–1006.

9. Botoman VA, Hanft KL, Breno SM, Vickers D, Astor FC, Caristo IB, Alemar GO, Sheth S, Bonner GF. Prospective controlled evaluation of pH testing, laryngoscopy and laryngopharyngeal sensory testing (LPST) shows a specific post inter-arytenoid neuropathy in proximal GERD (P-GERD). LPST improves laryngoscopy diagnostic yield in P-GERD. *Am J Gastroenterol.* 2002;97(9 suppl):S11–S12.

10. Leder SB, Ross DA, Briskin KB, Sasaki CT. A prospective, double-blind, randomized study on the use of a topical anesthetic, vasoconstrictor, and placebo during transnasal flexible fiberoptic endoscopy. *J Speech Lang Hear Res.* 1997;40:1352–1357.

11. Wyke B. Effects of anesthesia upon intrinsic laryngeal reflexes: an experimental study. *J Laryngol Otol.* 1968;82:603–612.

12. Murakami Y, Kirchner JA. Mechanical and physiologic properties of reflex laryngeal closure. *Ann Otol Rhinol Laryngol.* 1972;81:59–71.

13. Olsson GL, Hallen D Laryngospasm during anesthesia: a computer-aided incidence study in 136,929 patients. *Acta Anesthesiol Scand.* 1984;28:567–575.

14. Boushey HA, Richardson PS, Widdicombe JG, Wise JC. The response of laryngeal afferent fibres to mechanical and chemical stimuli. *J Physiol.* 1974;240:153–175.

15. Krouse HJ, Williams RC. Medical emergencies in office-based surgery. In: Krouse JH, Mirante JP, Christmas DA, eds. *Office-Based Surgery in Otolaryngology*. Philadelphia, Pa: WB Saunders; 1999:245–256.

16. Fox EJ, Sklar GS, Hill CH, Villanueva R, King BD. Complications related to the pressor response to endotracheal intubation. *Anesthesiology*. 1977;47:524–525.

17. Ovassapian A, Yelich SJ, Dykes MHM, Brunner EE. Blood pressure and heart rate changes during awake fiberoptic nasotracheal intubation. *Anesth Analg*. 1983;62:951–954.

18. Younger DS, Lange DJ, Lovelace RE, Blitzer A. Neuromuscular disorders of the larynx. In: Blitzer A, Brin MF, Sasaki CT, Fahn S, Harris KS, eds. *Neurologic Disorders of the Larynx*. New York, NY: Thieme Medical Publishers; 1992:240–247.

VII

Coding

1. FLEXIBLE ENDOSCOPIC EVALUATION OF SWALLOWING WITH SENSORY TESTING (FEESST), SENSORY TESTING, AND FIBEROPTIC ENDOSCOPIC EVALUATION OF SWALLOWING (FEES)

Introduction

FEESST, sensory testing, and FEES are relatively new procedures. The procedure codes for each are presented in this chapter, as is a history of the evolution of the coding for endoscopy for swallowing. Knowledge of the history behind the coding provides a perspective for clinicians as to how insurance carriers regard each of these procedures. Understanding the evolution of these codes helps prepare clinicians for the inevitable changes that will occur.

History of FEESST Current Procedural Terminology (CPT) Coding

There has been a considerable evolution in the CPT coding of FEESST, which has resulted in an increasing sophistication among the largest insurance carriers with respect to endoscopy for swallowing evaluations. As a result, coding for the various endoscopy procedures for swallowing has become much more precise. Prior to 1998, there were no CPT codes for FEESST, sensory testing, or fiberoptic endoscopic evaluation of swallowing (FEES). In 1998, Empire Medicare, the New York State Medicare carrier, issued the first codes for FEESST. At that time, Empire Medicare required three different codes for FEESST:

> 31575: Transnasal Flexible Laryngoscopy
>
> 92525: Swallowing Evaluation
>
> 92520-59: Laryngeal Function Studies

Note that a -59 modifier had to be used when specifically coding for FEESST. The -59 modifier signifies the following:

Under certain circumstances, the physician may need to indicate that a procedure or service was distinct or independent from other services performed on the same day. Modifier "-59" is used to identify procedures/services that are not normally reported together, but are appropriate under the circumstances.[1]

In the past, when a FEES was performed the codes needed were 31575 and 92525. When a laryngopharyngeal sensory test alone was performed, 92520-59 was supposed to be used. These codes were in place through January 31, 2002. However, on January 1, 2001, one year before the three aforementioned codes stopped being used, the Center for Medicaid and Medicare Services (CMS) introduced a new set of endoscopy for swallowing codes called "G-codes." The G-codes were a set of temporary codes to be used by clinicians until CMS, working with both the American Academy of Otolaryngology—Head and Neck Surgery (AAO–HNS) and the American Speech-Language-Hearing Association (ASHA), came up with a definitive set of codes for the "suite" of endoscopy for swallowing codes. One of the most important by-products of this combined effort was to assign, for the first time, relative value units (RVUs) to the endoscopy for swallowing code groups.

RVUs

RVUs differ depending on where the procedure is performed. Is the procedure performed in a "facility"—hospital, endoscopy suite, or operating room—or in a nonfacility—a physician's office? In general, the RVUs in a facility are almost always less than the RVUs in a nonfacility. The reason for this is that practice expense reimbursement is included in the RVU for procedures performed in a physician's office, but not when the procedure is performed in the hospital where it is assumed the hospital or the facility pays for the practice expenses (eg, gauze pads, cotton-tipped applicators, medications, etc).

CPT Codes for Endoscopy for Swallowing

The net results of these years of code evolution are the current endoscopy for swallowing codes, effective as of January 1, 2004. These codes (92612-92617) were first reported in the 2004 CPT manual and are explained in Table 7–1.

Nonfacility Endoscopy for Swallowing Codes

Table 7–2 lists the facility and nonfacility (physician's office) RVUs for the endoscopy for swallowing codes. To put these RVUs in perspective, the 2005 nonfacility (physician's office) RVU for transnasal flexible laryngoscopy (TFL) (31575) is 3.09, while the facility RVU for TFL is 2.08.

Table 7–1. CPT codes for endoscopy for swallowing

92612	Flexible fiberoptic endoscopic evaluation of swallowing **by cine or video recording;**
92613	with physician interpretation and report
92614	Flexible fiberoptic endoscopic evaluation, laryngeal sensory testing **by cine or video recording;**
92615	with physician interpretation and report
92616	Flexible fiberoptic endoscopic evaluation of swallowing and laryngeal sensory testing **by cine or video recording;**
92617	with physician interpretation and report

Table 7–2. 2005 RVUs for the endoscopy for swallowing codes for both nonfacility (NF) and facility (F).

	NF	F
FEES (92612)	**4.05**	**1.97**
Physician interpretation and report (**92613**)	**1.16**	**1.15**
Total FEES with		
Physician interpretation and report (92612 + 92613) =	**5.21**	**3.12**
Sensory Testing (92614)	**3.81**	**1.97**
Physician interpretation and report (92615)	**1.03**	**1.03**
Total sensory testing with		
Physician interpretation and report (92614 + 92615) =	**4.84**	**3.00**
FEESST 92616	**5.33**	**2.93**
Physician interpretation and report (**92617**)	**1.28**	**1.28**
Total FEESST with		
Physician interpretation and report (92616 + 92617) =	**6.61**	**4.21**

To begin to bring the RVUs into the realities of practice and to obtain an idea of what the reimbursement might be, the RVU is multiplied by a conversion factor that has local, regional, and national variations.

Video Record of the FEESST

There are several important points to be drawn from the CPT codes associated with FEESST, FEES, and sensory testing. First, the genesis of some of the wording of the latest endoscopy for swallowing codes stems from the CMS concern about their members not receiving the most comprehensive examination possible, hence the inclusion of the term *"by cine or video recording"* when describing the suite of endoscopy for swallowing codes. A clinician cannot simply insert a flexible endoscope through the nose, look through the laryngoscope eyepiece, ask the patient to drink some water, and call that a FEES examination. By insisting that the examination be recorded on either analog or digital media, CMS ensures some level of examination consistency. Now, to be reimbursed, the clinician must have a moving image record of the examination. This not only ensures some degree of relative consistency from examination to examination, but also is educational for the patient. The examination can be reviewed while the patient is still in the office or at the patient's bedside. In this way, the patient can see exactly what is happening with his or her swallow patterns. Furthermore, the clinician can make recommendations at the time of the exam. Additionally, with the majority of swallow action taking place in about 1 second, things are happening too fast for the clinician to make a specific diagnosis without first reviewing the filmed endoscopic procedure. At times, a frame-by-frame review is necessary to make the diagnosis. For example, if one sees pooled secretions in the piriform sinus, the question arises: Did the secretions come from above—meaning from the mouth—or were they regurgitated from below—meaning from the esophagus? A frame-by-frame review of the recorded endoscopic swallowing evaluation often answers this question. Also, with a separate code for physician interpretation and review of the taped exam, "swallowologists" can now follow the precedent in other fields of medicine in which clinicians receive reimbursement for reviewing and interpreting images. As a result, when the inevitable request for review of a tape of a patient's endoscopic swallowing evaluation comes into the physician's office ("Doctor, can you look at this tape for me and tell me what's going on?"), as of January 1, 2004, physicians can get reimbursed for their efforts.

ICD-9 Codes

In order for CPT codes to allow reimbursement for FEESST, FEES, and sensory testing, specific diagnostic or ICD-9 codes must be used. The appropriate diagnostic codes for the swallowing suite of codes are listed in Table 7–3. If one must remember a single ICD-9 code, it would be 787.2 or dysphagia.

TABLE 7-3. Diagnostic codes compatible with the endoscopy for swallowing CPT codes

Code	Description
150.0	Malignant neoplasm of cervical esophagus
150.1	Malignant neoplasm of thoracic esophagus
150.2	Malignant neoplasm of abdominal esophagus
150.3	Malignant neoplasm of upper third of esophagus
150.4	Malignant neoplasm of middle third of esophagus
150.5	Malignant neoplasm of lower third of esophagus
150.8	Malignant neoplasm of esophagus, other specified part
150.9	Malignant neoplasm of esophagus, unspecified
235.6	Neoplasm of uncertain behavior of larynx
239.1	Neoplasms of unspecified nature, respiratory system
332.0	Paralysis agitans
332.1	Secondary Parkinsonism
333.0	Other degenerative diseases of the basal ganglia
333.2	Myoclonus
333.4	Huntington's chorea
333.5	Other choreas
333.6	Idiopathic torsion dystonia
333.81	Fragments of torsion dystonia, blepharospasm
333.82	Fragments of torsion dystonia, orofacial dyskinesia
333.83	Fragments of torsion dystonia, spasmodic torticollis
333.84	Fragments of torsion dystonia, organic writers' cramp
333.89	Fragments of torsion dystonia, other
333.90	Other and unspecified extrapyramidal diseases and abnormal movement disorder
333.91	Other and unspecified extrapyramidal diseases and abnormal movement disorder, stiff-man syndrome
333.92	Other and unspecified extrapyramidal diseases and abnormal movement disorder, neuroleptic malignant syndrome
333.93	Other and unspecified extrapyramidal diseases and abnormal movement disorder, benign shuddering attacks
333.99	Other and unspecified extrapyramidal diseases and abnormal movement disorder, other
335.20	Amyotrophic lateral sclerosis

continues

TABLE 7–3. *continued*

Code	Description
341.0	Neuromyelitis optica
341.1	Schilder's disease
341.8	Other demyelinating diseases of central nervous system
341.9	Demyelinating diseases of central nervous system, unspecified
342.00	Flaccid hemiplegia, affecting unspecified side
342.01	Flaccid hemiplegia, affecting dominant side
342.02	Flaccid hemiplegia, affecting nondominant side
342.10	Spastic hemiplegia, affecting unspecified side
342.11	Spastic hemiplegia, affecting dominant side
342.12	Spastic hemiplegia, affecting nondominant side
342.80	Other specified hemiplegia, affecting unspecified side
342.81	Other specified hemiplegia, affecting dominant side
342.82	Other specified hemiplegia, affecting nondominant side
342.90	Hemiplegia, unspecifed, affecting unspecified side
342.91	Hemiplegia, unspecifed, affecting dominant side
342.92	Hemiplegia, unspecifed, affecting nondominant side
436	Acute, but ill-defined, cerebrovascular disease
438.10	Speech and language deficit, unspecified
438.11	Aphasia
438.12	Dysphasia
438.19	Other speech and language deficits
438.20	Hemiplegia affecting unspecified side
438.21	Hemiplegia affecting dominant side
438.22	Hemiplegia affecting nondominant side
438.50	Other paralytic syndrome affecting unspecified side
438.51	Other paralytic syndrome affecting dominant side
438.52	Other paralytic syndrome affecting nondominant side
438.53	Other paralytic syndrome, bilateral
438.82	Dysphagia, cerebrovascular disease
438.83	Facial weakness/Facial droop
464.01	Acute laryngitis with obstruction
464.51	Supraglottis, unspecified with obstruction

continues

TABLE 7–3. *continued*

Code	Description
478.30	Paralysis of vocal cords or larynx, paralysis, unspecified
478.31	Paralysis of vocal cords or larynx, unilateral, partial
478.32	Paralysis of vocal cords or larynx, unilateral, complete
478.33	Paralysis of vocal cords or larynx, bilateral, partial
478.34	Paralysis of vocal cords or larynx, bilateral, complete
478.6	Edema of larynx
507.0	Pneumonitis due to solids and liquids, due to inhalation of food or vomitus
530.0	Achalasia and cardiospasm
530.20	Ulcer of esophagus without bleeding
530.21	Ulcer of esophagus with bleeding
530.3	Stricture and stenosis of esophagus
530.6	Diverticulum of esophagus, acquired
530.81	Esophageal reflux
530.85	Barrett's esophagus
783.3	Feeding difficulties and mismanagement
787.2	Dysphagia
933.1	Foreign body in larynx
934.0 -934.9	Food or foreign body in trachea, bronchus or lung
V48.3	Mechanical and motor problems with neck and trunk

2. TRANSNASAL ESOPHAGOSCOPY (TNE)

One of the most telling reasons we believe esophagoscopy will be performed more and more routinely in an office setting comes from an analysis of the RVUs for TNE (Table 7–4). Because of the previously discussed risks of conscious sedation, and the even greater risks with general anesthesia, the costs of performing esophagoscopy in a facility are far greater than the costs of performing esophagoscopy in an office setting without sedation. TNE encompasses what we believe will be the future of office-based procedures: safer for patients, less lost work time for patients, and enhanced practice efficiency for physicians.

Table 7-4. 2005 CPT codes and RVUs for transnasal esophagoscopy (TNE) for both nonfacility (NF) and facility (F).

	NF	F
43200 Esophagoscopy, rigid or flexible; diagnostic	5.85	2.79
43202 Esophagoscopy, rigid or flexible; with biopsy, single or multiple	7.59	2.99

3. PANENDOSCOPY (LARYNGOSCOPY WITH BIOPSY AND ESOPHAGOSCOPY WITH OR WITHOUT BIOPSY)

During the course of a sensory test or a FEESST, a mass may be found in the laryngopharynx that may require further investigation, in particular, laryngopharyngeal biopsy and an endoscopic investigation of the esophagus, or panendoscopy. Although the true definition of an upper aerodigestive tract panendoscopy means an endoscopic examination of the laryngopharynx, lungs, and esophagus, in current parlance, panendoscopy practically means laryngoscopy and esophagoscopy. Most adult bronchoscopies today are being performed by pulmonologists. TNE technology allows the physician and the patient to have their endoscopic examinations of the laryngopharynx and esophagus in the physician's office instead of the operating room. The advantages to performing panendoscopy in the office, and thereby avoiding the operating room, are:

1. Avoiding endotracheal intubation.
2. Avoiding general anesthesia.
3. Saving operating room time because the typical time it can take for a panendoscopy under general anesthesia is roughly 2 hours.
4. Enhancing practice efficiency because the same 2-hour period of operating room time can be reduced to about 30 minutes to perform in the office (Table 7–5).

In a practice situation where an otolaryngologist has three pandendoscopies scheduled for a particular day, one can quickly see the advantage of performing these procedures in the office. Instead of spending 6 hours performing three rigid laryngoscopies and three

Table 7-5. 2005 CPT codes and RVUs for panendoscopy (laryngoscopy with biopsy and esophagoscopy) for both non-facility (NF) and facility (F).

PANENDOSCOPY IN OPERATING ROOM (F)	
31535 Direct Laryngoscopy and biopsy	5.41
43200 Esophagoscopy, rigid or flexible; diagnostic	2.79
TOTAL:	**7.20**
or	
31535 Direct Laryngoscopy and biopsy	5.41
43202 Esophagoscopy, rigid or flexible; with biopsy, single or multiple	2.9
TOTAL:	**8.40**
PANENDOSCOPY IN OFFICE (NF)	
31576 TFL & biopsy	5.78
43200 Esophagoscopy, rigid or flexible; diagnostic	5.85
TOTAL	**11.63**
or	
31576 TFL & biopsy	5.78
43202 Esophagoscopy, rigid or flexible; with biopsy, single or multiple	7.59
TOTAL	**13.37**

rigid esophagoscopies, with in-office TFL and biopsy and TNE with or without biopsy, the physician requires only 90 minutes on the same set of procedures (Table 7–5). More importantly, the three patients who would have undergone general endotracheal anesthesia with its attendant risks and loss of an entire day of work or play now are able to walk out of the office and immediately resume their lives.

4. SUMMARY

This chapter presents the current state of coding for endoscopy for swallowing and TNE. Because codes and RVUs may change in the future, it is up to the clinician to keep track of the inevitable changes that will occur while at the same time always being careful to use the codes appropriately.

REFERENCES

1. American Medical Association. *CPT "98: Physicians" Current Procedural Terminology.* Chicago, Ill: AMA; 1998.

VIII

Cases

In this chapter, several cases are presented to illustrate the FEESST directed, decision-making process. Although no two patients are exactly alike, the cases we present are derived from diagnostic categories most likely to have swallowing disorders. As will be seen in each case, the importance of a thorough history prior to any testing is imperative regardless of the primary complaint. This is especially true in patients who have multiple complaints or whose complaints are not well described. Conditions at the onset, family history, current and past medicines taken, previous diagnoses, and types of treatment tried are all part of the workup prior to testing.

1. CASE 1: PARKINSON'S DISEASE

Description

> A 56-year-old male attorney with a 3-year history of Parkinson's disease was referred by his neurologist because his voice had become noticeably weaker in the past 7 months following an upper respiratory infection (URI). He reported a change in his voice coinciding with the diagnosis of Parkinson's, but it had remained stable until 7 months ago. Since then, he has noticed an increase in throat clearing, excess mucus, globus sensation, and increased cough. On further questioning, he noted that the cough was more pronounced after eating lunch and dinner.

On the GRBAS perceptual voice assessment scale, he was G = 2, R = 1, B = 2, A = 2, S = 1.[1] The GRBAS Scale was developed especially for clinicians to scale the severity of the voice based on perceptual features. The scale ranges from 0 (not present) to 4 (severe).

G = Grade—an overall rating of severity

R = Roughness—the degree of rough voice quality

B = Breathiness—the degree of excess breath flow in the voice

A = Asthenic—the degree of weakness in the voice

S = Strain or spasm—the degree of strain or tightness in the voice

His Reflux Symptom Index (RSI)[2] was 27, and his 10-question voice handicap index (VHI-10) was 23.[3] He did not complain of heartburn or regurgitation. His wife indicated that he had lost approximately 6 pounds since the URI. Over the past 6 months, his pharmacologic profile has been relatively stable and includes Sinemet, Lipitor, 81 mg aspirin, Elavil, and a multivitamin.

Based on his symptoms of voice change, dysphagia, and coughing after meals, a FEESST examination was done. Once the endoscope was in place, velopharyngeal closure was assessed to be normal. The vocal folds were mobile and had no lesions. There was also pseudosulcus vocalis, arytenoid and interarytenoid edema, and thick mucus in the piriform sinuses, epiglottis, and arytenoids. The sensory test results showed the laryngeal adductor reflex (LAR) was elicited bilaterally at 7.2 mm Hg air pulse pressure. The laryngeal squeeze was tested with high-pitch phonation and was felt to be intact. When given a teaspoon of applesauce to swallow, there was no penetration or aspiration; but there was diffuse residual bolus in the hypopharynx after each swallow (Fig 8–1). The patient was given water to swallow (liquid washdown), which resulted in near total clearing of the residual bolus (Fig 8–2).

Based on the symmetric reduced laryngopharyngeal sensation recorded during the sensory testing, and the pseudosulcus and interarytenoid edema, a diagnosis of laryngopharyngeal reflux (LPR) was made and the patient was placed on a proton pump inhibitor (PPI) 30 to 60 minutes before breakfast and dinner. He was also instructed to add a 300-milliliter (ml) nutritional supplement to his daily diet and, when eating his meals, to follow solids with a sip of water ("liquid washdown"). He was also told to monitor his weight every week and bring the results with him on the next visit. A return visit was scheduled in 3 months. He expressed great relief when the examination was over, because he indicated that based on what he had read about Parkinson's disease, he was worried that he would need to be placed on percutaneous endoscopic gastrostomy (PEG) feeding. When he returned 3 months later for a follow-up examination, his RSI was down to 16 and his VHI-10 was down to 13, still above normal. His voice was weak with mild dysarthria. At this visit, his primary complaint was a weak voice at the end of the day. His coughing during and after eating was reduced but not completely eliminated. His weight remained stable

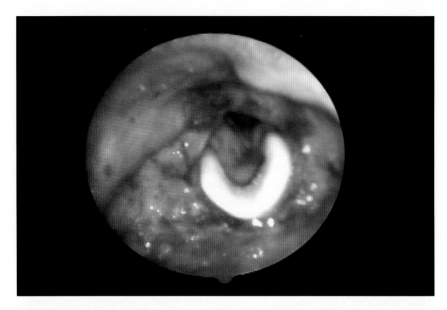

FIGURE 8–1. Case 1 (Parkinson's disease). Residual food in hypopharynx during a FEESST. There is a copious amount of green-laden pureed food material throughout laryngopharynx.

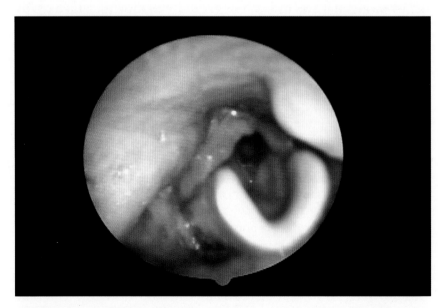

FIGURE 8–2. Case 1 (Parkinson's disease). Clearance of pooled secretions after liquid washdown. In the same patient shown in Figure 8-1, note how most of the green material has now been cleared away from the hypopharynx subsequent to drinking a clear liquid.

over the 3-month period. The sensory test was repeated and it revealed a bilateral mild sensory deficit of 5.7 mm Hg air pulse pressure. He was referred for Lee Silverman Voice Treatment and asked to remain on PPI therapy until his return in 6 months.

Interpretation

In most cases of Parkinson's, swallowing and speech continually degrade. However, if the patient has the opportunity to continue working and remain active, rehabilitation in the form of medical treatment, swallowing therapy, and voice building using the Lee Silverman Voice Treatment program should be made available. A 4- to 6-month follow-up schedule is appropriate for the above patient. What the FEESST enabled the clinicians to do was to maximize the types and amounts of foods the patient could safely tolerate so that he could sustain himself on oral intake alone. In addition, the contribution of sensory deficits from the patient's reflux disease could be directly assessed and the progress of antacid therapy—and its effect on swallowing function—could be closely followed.

2. CASE 2: VASCULAR MALFORMATION

Description

A healthy 28-year-old female pediatric nurse with three episodes of aspiration pneumonia over a 9-month period was seen in the office for further evaluation. Although she experienced no weight loss, she was concerned about her recurring bouts of pneumonia. She was being followed by a pulmonologist who diagnosed bronchiectasis in the right mainstem bronchus, possibly of viral etiology. She reported no dysphagia or odynophagia, and she was a nonsmoker. Her RSI was 19, abnormal; and her VHI-10 was 4, suggesting normal voice.

She was referred for FEESST by her pulmonologist following a modified barium swallow (MBS) that was reportedly normal with no evidence of penetration or aspiration on liquids, puree, or a cookie.

On the transnasal flexible laryngoscopy (TFL) portion of her laryngopharyngeal sensory test, her vocal folds were normal and showed symmetric abduction and adduction. Her voice was normal in pitch and voice quality and her GRBAS score was G = 1, R = 0, B = 0, A = 0, S = 1. On sensory testing, a severe right sensory deficit was found (8.8 mm Hg air pulse pressure). Sensation on the left was determined to be 3.4 mm Hg air pulse pressure, which is within normal limits. Her swallowing of liquids, puree, and a cookie was normal. Because the sensory testing showed an asymmetry of response to air pulse stimulation, a magnetic resonance imaging (MRI) of the brain and neck was ordered. A 9-centimeter (cm), left supratentorial vascular malformation was identified. The patient was immediately referred for neurological surgery consultation.

Interpretation

This case is a great example of how sensory testing alone can be used to assess the integrity of the sensory component of the vagus nerve. In most instances when a patient presents with a history of unexplained pneumonia, a TFL alone would be performed. However, a TFL alone or even a fiberoptic endoscopic examination of swallowing (FEES) alone likely would have missed the laryngopharyngeal sensory asymmetry, which would have wasted valuable time as potentially serious disease progression continued.

3. CASE 3: NEURALGIA

Description

A 58-year-old businessman was referred by his gastrointestinal (GI) doctor for evaluation of mild hoarseness and a persistent "burning throat." The patient described a 9-month history of intermittent, intense burning in the throat and upper chest, which occasionally radiated to his right ear lobule. He noted no change in weight for the past year. He quit smoking 35 years ago; prior to that time, he was a one pack per day smoker for approximately 6 years. An esophagogastroduodenoscopy (EGD) done shortly after the onset of the burning revealed a hiatal hernia; and as a result of the EGD, he was placed on a PPI. After 8 weeks of PPI therapy, the patient had no resolution of his throat burning complaint despite the fact that he stopped eating chocolate and reduced his intake of caffeine and citrus foods. The patient also noted frequent throat clearing, cough, excess phlegm, and occasional weakness in his voice. A computed tomography (CT) scan of the neck obtained by his internist was unremarkable. Because of persistent burning in his throat, he was referred for consultation to our Voice and Swallowing Center.

His RSI was 11, and his VHI-10 was 0. A head and neck examination was done. There were no palpable masses in the neck and no asymmetry in facial expression. A laryngopharyngeal sensory test was performed. The vocal folds were visualized and showed pseudosulcus vocalis, posterior commissure hypertrophy, and a small granuloma on the left posterior vocal process. There was symmetry of vocal fold abduction on the "eeee, sniff" task. When stimulated with the air pulse, he showed a severe unilateral sensory deficit of 9.1 mm Hg air pulse pressure on the right side and normal sensation of 3.4 mm Hg air pulse pressure on the left side. The diagnosis was a right superior laryngeal nerve neuralgia, and laryngopharyngeal reflux disease with a vocal process granuloma. His antacid medicine was increased to twice daily, 30 to 60 minutes before breakfast and dinner, and 150 mg of ranitidine at bedtime was added as well. He was referred for an MRI with gadolinium of the brain to rule out a mass in the right brainstem. He was also advised to see a neurologist with specialization in pain management.

On follow-up examination 2 months later, the patient noted a reduction of the throat "burning" and less coughing. His RSI was 10, and his VHI-10 remained at 0. He saw the neurologist who started him on 300 mg neurontin, which was escalated to 1200 mg per day over a 6-week period. His MRI did not reveal any mass along the course of the vagus nerve. Repeat sensory testing on that visit continued to show a right unilateral, severe sensory deficit and normal sensation on the left. Because he continued to have throat clearing and excess mucus, a session of vocal hygiene was ordered, as was a consultation with a registered dietician.

On a follow-up visit 2 months later, the patient indicated that his throat burning was beginning to subside. His neurontin dosage was now decreased to 600 mg per day, and he was experiencing only rare throat clearing. His RSI was 5, and his VHI-10 remained at 0. His reflux medicine was reduced to once daily and a 6-month follow-up evaluation and sensory test was recommended.

Interpretation

When the primary complaint from the patient is "burning," we are immediately alerted to the possible diagnosis of some type of vagal nerve neuralgia, because dysphagia and LPR symptoms rarely include burning in the throat as a complaint. Coupling the patient's symptom of burning with the sign of an asymmetric laryngopharyngeal sensory deficit led to the diagnosis of SLN neuralgia. Even when a patient also has strong evidence of LPR as an additional diagnosis, he or she often needs neurontin as well as PPI therapy to effectively treat the complaint.

4. CASE 4: STROKE

Description

A 72-year-old salesman presented to the hospital emergency room with acute onset of dysphagia, drooling, coughing, hoarseness, and a right hemiparesis. Neurologic workup, including an MRI of the brain, revealed a right brainstem stroke.

The patient underwent a FEESST, and the laryngeal exam was notable for decreased abduction of the right true vocal fold, right vocal fold bowing, and significant arytenoid and interarytenoid edema (Fig 8–3). The sensory test revealed a severe sensory deficit on the right with the laryngeal adductor reflex (LAR) elicited only on

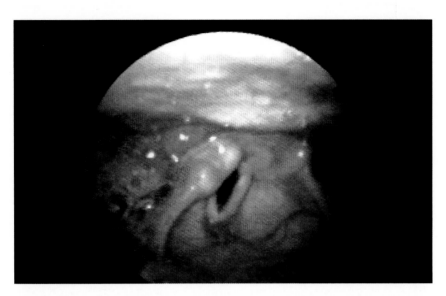

FIGURE 8–3. Case 4 (Stroke). Pooling of food in right piriform sinus during a FEESST. There is a heap of green-colored food sitting in the right piriform sinus. In addition, the right vocal fold is bowed and the right arytenoid appears pulled anteriorly. Arytenoid and interarytenoid edema and ventricle obliteration are also visible.

continuous air pulse stimulation and normal sensation on the left with the LAR elicited at 3.5 mm Hg air pulse pressure. During the food administration portion of the FEESST, there was pooling of secretions and food in the right piriform sinus, laryngeal penetration, and trace aspiration of thin liquids with immediate cough observed. Thick liquids were tolerated without laryngeal penetration. Turning the head to the right resulted in resolution of the right piriform pooling.

As a result of the FEESST, the plan of treatment included thickened liquids, head turn to the right, and throat clearing after each thick liquid swallow. A proton pump inhibitor was also prescribed, to be taken 30 to 60 minutes before breakfast. In addition, a referral to a dietitian was made for a calorie count and dietary management. A follow-up FEESST performed 3 months later revealed a 3-pound weight gain and minor improvement in sensation (8.5 mm Hg air pulse pressure on right). Thin liquid swallow revealed slight penetration that was cleared immediately with a cough. The treatment plan was then modified to begin taking thin liquids followed by a cough. Dietary and pharmacologic treatments were maintained for an additional 3 months.

Interpretation

When evaluating dysphagia in a patient with a stroke, obtaining the sensory information afforded during a FEESST allows the clinician to apply behavioral management techniques very precisely. Moreover, because stroke can affect not only the central efferent, or motor, control systems, but the afferent, or sensory, control systems as well, a FEESST enables the clinician to address both of these interrelated systems.

5. CASE 5: LARYNGOPHARYNGEAL REFLUX (LPR)

Description

> A 52-year-old female librarian with hoarseness for 2 years that had increased over the past 5 months was referred by her primary care physician. The patient is a lifetime non-smoker with intermittent complaints of dysphagia and rare episodes of heartburn. On presentation, she is noted to be morbidly obese presenting with cough, hoarseness, throat clearing, and excess phlegm.

A laryngopharyngeal sensory test was performed. When the larynx was visualized, an irregular mass was noted on the left vocal process (Fig 8–4A). The vocal folds showed slightly decreased abduction on the left side. Sensory testing revealed bilateral symmetric severe sensory deficits with the LAR elicited at 9.0 mm Hg air pulse pressure. The food administration trials of the FEEEST revealed no penetration on any of the administered food consistencies. She was placed on PPI therapy twice daily, referred to the voice therapist near her home, and given instructions on vocal hygiene that included increasing her water intake, reducing her intake of caffeine, chocolate, alcohol, and mints and given instruction on the silent cough technique to reduce throat clearing. The silent cough technique consists of a thrust of air from the lungs without

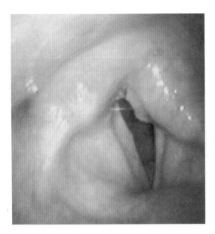 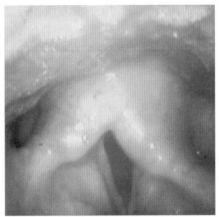

A.   **B.**

FIGURE 8–4. Case 5 (LPR). A. Left arytenoid granuloma. Endoscopic
view of laryngopharynx of patient at initial FEESST demonstrating a left arytenoid granuloma and edema of arytenoids. **B. Resolution of left arytenoid granuloma.** Endoscopic appearance of larynx after a 3-month
course of a proton pump inhibitor. Note resolution of the left arytenoid
granuloma, and subjective improvement in arytenoid edema.

closing the mouth. The vocal folds do not approximate, there is only the sound of air rushing out of the mouth but the persistent mucus is blown away from the vocal folds and airway. Following the
thrust of air, the patient is also instructed to swallow. Eventually
the throat clearing habit is replaced with a simple swallow.

   She returned 3 months later after completing eight sessions of
voice therapy and reported medication compliance of 90%. Repeat
flexible endoscopic examination of the laryngopharynx revealed
resolution of the left vocal process mass (Fig 8–4B). Sensory testing
was now found to be near normal bilaterally (4.5 mg Hg air pulse
pressure). Her PPI medication was reduced to once per day in the
morning 30 minutes before breakfast and she was given a follow-
up appointment for 4 months.

Interpretation

In patients with bilateral, symmetric, severe sensory deficits, where
there is no history of neurologic disease or stroke, LPR alone must
be considered in the differential diagnosis of the etiology of the patient's complaints [4.]

6. CASE 6: DYSPHAGIA FOLLOWING OPEN-HEART SURGERY

Description

> A 58-year-old male physician referred from the open-heart
> intensive care unit (ICU) was seen 4 days status post aortic
> valve replacement. He complained of difficulty swallowing
> solid foods and liquids since extubation on postoperative
> day 2. When the patient was given some food, he coughed
> so he was placed on nasogastric tube feedings and not per-
> mitted to take food by mouth. From a cardiac perspective,
> the patient was hemodynamically stable, ready to be dis-
> charged from the ICU. However, the ICU staff was con-
> cerned about the patient's inability to swallow, so a FEESST
> was requested.

Endoscopic examination of the larynx revealed bilateral vocal
fold granulomas (Fig 8–5). The sensory portion of the FEESST
showed a bilateral severe laryngopharyngeal sensory deficit with
the LAR elicited only on continuous air stimulation. The pharyngeal squeeze was intact. During the food administration trials, there
was slight aspiration of thin liquids, which was cleared immediately. Purees, mechanical soft, and honey and nectar-thickened liquids
were tolerated without laryngeal penetration. The patient was
placed on a diet consisting of mechanical soft food with nectar-
thickened liquids. In addition, PPI therapy, twice a day, taken 30 to
60 minutes before breakfast and dinner was recommended.
Avoiding caffeine, chocolate, alcohol, and mint was also suggested,
as was good oral hygiene and a calorie count. With these instructions, the patient was discharged from the ICU and 1 week later discharged from the hospital on the aforementioned modified diet.

Interpretation

This case represents what we have been seeing in greater and
greater numbers in the past 5 years, namely, dysphagia after open-

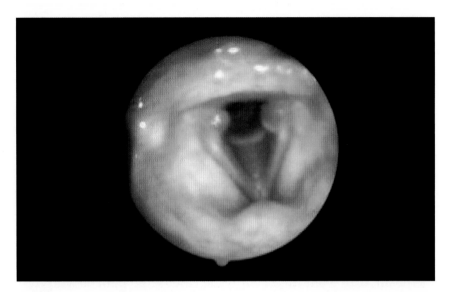

FIGURE 8–5. Case 6 (after open-heart surgery). Bilateral arytenoid granulomas. In this endoscopic view of the laryngopharynx, note the two epithelial protuberances along the vocal processes of the arytenoids, which are granulomas.

heart surgery. The causes are multifactorial; but when a neurologic event is ruled out, we believe that untreated or insufficiently treated laryngopharyngeal reflux disease must be considered a likely cause in the differential diagnosis.

7. SUMMARY

Laryngopharyngeal sensory testing, whether utilized as a stand-alone test or as part of a FEESST examination, has direct, crucial application in the management of a variety of very common disease processes, such as acid reflux disease, stroke, and chronic neurodegenerative disease. In addition, less common, but very vexing, disease entities such as central vascular malformations and vagal nerve neuralgia can be more readily detected when laryngopharyngeal sensory testing is applied in the workup of the swallowing problems that can be manifested as a consequence of these disease processes. Very often, the only hint that neuralgia or a process producing some sort of central mass effect is the etiology of the patient's dysphagia complaint is an asymmetric laryngopharyngeal sensory test. Finally, the dysphagia sequellae of open-heart surgery on an ever-aging population will likely loom large as a very common source of requests for inpatient dysphagia consultation. Consequently, FEESST, with its emphasis on assessment of airway protection, is an essential component of the diagnosis and treatment of this cohort of patients. Our hope, and the way we have been assessing patients with dysphagia, is that attention to the sensory component of swallowing ultimately will carry the same clinical weight as the assessment of the motor component of swallowing.

Laryngopharyngeal sensory testing and FEESST allow both patients with dysphagia and the various physician specialists taking care of them the opportunity for comprehensive diagnosis and management in the office setting. Sending the patient with a swallowing complaint out of the office for an essential diagnostic test of swallowing will soon be increasingly infrequent. FEESST also gives the health care team involved in the care of the patient with dysphagia the option of being present during the discovery of the source of the swallowing problem and testing of the therapeutic maneuvers that might be applied to assist the patient in swallowing more safely.

As a result of the amalgamation of immediate in-office assessment, the application of sensory and motor information, and real-time viewing of the dysphagia problem and its possible solutions, there will be greater continuity of care and greater likelihood of successful treatment for the patient with dysphagia.

REFERENCES

1. Hirano M. *Clinical Examination of the Voice.* New York, NY: Springer; 1981.
2. Belafsky PC, Postma GN, Koufman JA. Validity and reliability of the reflux symptom index (RSI). *J Voice.* 2002;16:274–277.
3. Rosen CA, Lee AS, Osborne J, Zullo T, Murry T. Development and validation of the Voice Handicap Index-10. *Laryngoscope.* 2004;114:1549–1556.
4. Aviv JE, Liu H, Parides M, Kaplan ST, Close LG. Laryngopharyngeal sensory deficits in patients with laryngopharyngeal reflux and dysphagia. *Ann Otol Rhinol Laryngol* 2000; 109:1000-1006.

Index